Practical Intervention for
Cleft Palate Speech

Jane Russell & Liz Albery

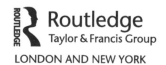

Routledge
Taylor & Francis Group

LONDON AND NEW YORK

Acknowledgements

We would like to thank the children, their parents and the adults with whom we have worked and who helped us to develop many of the therapy ideas and procedures outlined in this book. In addition we would like to acknowledge the contribution of our colleagues in the field, in particular Anne Harding-Bell and Alison Jeremy.

For the purposes of clarity alone, in this text 'he' is used to refer to the client, and 'she' to refer to the therapist.

First Published 2005 by Speechmark Publishing Ltd.

Published 2019 by Routledge
2 Park Square, Milton Park, Abingdon, Oxon OX14 4RN
52 Vanderbilt Avenue, New York, NY 10017

Routledge is an imprint of the Taylor & Francis Group, an informa business

British Library Cataloguing in Publication Data
Russell, Jane, 1951–
    Practical intervention for cleft palate speech. – (A Speechmark practical therapy resource)
    1. Cleft palate – Complications   2. Speech therapy
    I. Title   II. Albery, E. H.
    617.5'225

ISBN: 978-0-86388-513-6 (pbk)

Contents

Figures & Tables

Figures

Tables

Handouts

Introduction

The provision of care in the UK

Over the past few years there have been major changes in the organisation of services in the UK to meet the needs of the child with cleft lip and palate or associated anomalies. In 1998, the government-sponsored Clinical Standards Advisory Group published a report (CSAG, 1998). The CSAG report found that standards of care in some units in the UK, particularly in facial growth outcomes, did not reach the same level as those provided in the best European centres (for example, Oslo). To address this it was recommended that far fewer centres undertake surgery for children and adults with cleft lip and palate so that the chosen centres would gather more numbers for audit and house a full complement of specialists to meet the needs of this population. Worldwide there are other examples of centres operating on too few cases, which results in less than optimal care for the child with a cleft.

In the UK this protracted and, for some, painful process is now virtually complete, with a total of 10 centres (excluding Scotland) undertaking primary surgery on a minimum of 80 new cases of cleft lip and/or palate per year. Within each centre highly-trained specialist speech and language therapists offer assessment and therapy for their population. They also network with link therapists in their region, who may attend local multidisciplinary clinics, undertake early screening and carry out a significant amount of therapy. It would be impractical for all therapy to be concentrated at the surgical centre, even though parents are prepared to travel for surgery a few times during childhood, regular speech therapy sessions (or orthodontic sessions) 50 or more miles from home would be an unreasonable burden. It is therefore important that a network of therapists who can acquire a level of specialism is attached to each surgical centre.

Developing specialist skills

It is hoped that this book goes some way towards addressing this need and equipping link and local therapists with the specialist skills that they need.

Experienced therapists will appreciate that when working with this client group there is an element of trial and error. What works well for one client may not work so well for another. We hope that the suggestions presented in this book will help the process of determining the best approach for a particular client. In addition, particularly when there is little progress, we recommend consulting the specialist speech and language therapists who work in the designated surgical centre cleft palate teams. This could be the therapist on the team involved with the particular client or one of the Royal College of Speech & Language Therapists (RCSLT) regional clinical advisers on cleft palate.

The aim of this book is to describe the role of the speech and language therapist and to provide practical ideas that can be incorporated into therapy programmes for use with clients whose speech difficulties arise from cleft palate and/or velopharyngeal disorders.

Origins and associated problems

Further information about the origin, incidence and nature of both overt and submucous clefts is provided by Albery and Russell (1990), McWilliams *et al* (1990) and Stengelhofen (1990). These texts also describe velopharyngeal insufficiency (VPI), which may occur with or without an associated cleft of the palate (Watson *et al*, 2001). The syndrome known as velocardiofacial or Di George syndrome is increasingly recognised and results from a missing piece of genetic information on the long arm of one of the twenty-second chromosomes. These syndromes are known as the 22q11 group and pose an additional challenge to the therapist in terms of management because, as well as an overt or submucous cleft palate, there may also be learning difficulties and behavioural issues that will affect therapy progress (Golding-Kushner, 2001).

It is self-evident that a physical defect affecting the structures of the mouth and face has the potential to influence communication and articulatory development in particular. In addition there may be associated hearing problems, particularly fluctuating conductive hearing loss resulting from otitis media (Albery & Russell, 1990). Children with cleft palate have been shown to be 'at risk' for developmental problems, especially delay in language development (Russell, 1989; Albery & Russell, 1990).

However, the majority of children who undergo primary surgery of the lip and/or palate in early childhood achieve normal speech and language skills. Management by the speech and language therapist is still required but takes the form of advice to the parents, together with the monitoring of communication development. This facilitates the early identification of delayed or deviant development and allows appropriate management to be implemented.

Using this book

The therapy ideas presented in this book should be used flexibly. They are designed to cover all age groups, including pre-school, school-aged and adult clients. Much of this book focuses on working with children, but Chapter 7 looks in particular at working with teenage and adult clients. We hope that therapists will take the ideas, expand them and incorporate them, as appropriate, into programmes that will meet the needs of individual clients. The primary focus in this book is on speech. If other communication skills need remediating, these should also be included in the therapy programme.

Planning Therapy

Principles of therapy

1 Comprehensive assessment and accurate diagnosis of the presenting speech disorder.
2 Identification of the aims of therapy and specific treatment goals.
3 Treatment tailored to the client's intellectual level, age, responsiveness and speech needs.
4 Intervention following operant learning principles, with the client as an active participant in the learning process.
5 Therapy should be structured and focused.

Assessment

The importance of undertaking a comprehensive assessment of all aspects of communication cannot be over-stressed. With young children in particular, the therapist must take an holistic approach and consider the whole child in relation to his environment rather than concentrate exclusively on the obvious physical defect. Factors relating to the structural abnormality should be taken into account, but these must not prevent the therapist from being open-minded until a differential diagnosis is reached.

Taking a case history

Children with a repaired cleft palate usually have a speech assessment at the age of 18 months/two years by a specialist speech and language therapist, followed by assessments at age three, five, 10 and 15 years (for audit as well as clinical purposes). However, a therapist working in the community may be asked to see a child with a repaired cleft palate or a child with an undiagnosed submucous cleft at any age. In addition to the information routinely obtained at an initial interview, there are some additional factors to consider when taking a case history. These include, where possible, the nature and extent of the original defect, and the timing and type of any operations. With young children it is also useful to obtain details about early feeding. Poor sucking or nasal regurgitation of milk during feeding are typical signs of velopharyngeal incompetence. Discussion during the taking of a case history helps the therapist to gain some insight into the parents'/carer's and/or client's understanding of the cleft palate condition (Russell, 1989). The results of hearing tests also provide essential information for the therapist. All children with cleft palate should, of course, be receiving regular hearing checks and the routine developmental screening that is carried out on all children.

Investigating the development of communication skills

Following the case history, the therapist will proceed with initial assessment, using informal and formal testing procedures to investigate all areas of communication development. With younger clients these will include play, non-verbal skills, verbal comprehension, vocabulary, syntax, semantics, articulation, phonetic and phonological development, and pragmatic skills. The methods of assessment are selected as appropriate for the age of the individual client. From the initial assessment the therapist will identify areas where further in-depth assessment is required.

The *Great Ormond Street Speech Assessment, GOS.SP.ASS*, (Sell *et al*, 1994, 1999) and Cleft Audit Protocol for Speech – Augmented, CAPS-A (John *et al*, in press) are screening procedures that have been developed specifically for describing the speech characteristics commonly associated with cleft palate and VPI. They are practical and time-efficient procedures that enable the therapist to identify speech characteristics requiring further investigation. In addition the procedure can be used to measure progress over time and facilitate comparison between different clients.

When the initial assessment indicates that there are specific speech problems, it is important to carry out a full phonetic and phonological analysis in addition to the oral examination and investigation of articulatory ability. Use of these types of analyses with cleft palate clients is described and illustrated in Albery and Russell (1990) and Grunwell (1993).

Oral examination

An oral examination should always be done on initial assessment as some speech characteristics may be explained by an obvious structural abnormality. There are comprehensive oral examination guidelines to be found in the Great Ormond Street Speech Assessment (GOS.SP.ASS, see Sell *et al*, 1994, 1999). If this is not available, the following features should be assessed. You will need a pen torch, disposable gloves and a disposable tongue depressor.

Face and head

Are there any dysmorphic features? For example, a relatively expressionless face or low cup-shaped ears associated with velocardiofacial syndrome (see page 2).

Lips

With current surgical techniques a repaired cleft lip is rarely immobile and bilabial sounds should not be affected, but if there is an underlying severe jaw malocclusion it may be difficult to obtain lip closure.

Teeth

Are there missing teeth in the line of the cleft, Class 3 malocclusion (usually due to undergrowth of the maxilla) or an anterior open bite? Any of these may affect the articulation of fricatives, such as /s/ in particular, or bilabial consonants.

Hard palate

Is the hard palate narrowed? This may restrict the normal tongue position for alveolar consonants. Is there a fistula? Many fistulae are very small and unlikely to affect speech, but occasionally they are responsible for nasal emission or, depending on their position, difficulty in articulating /t, d, s, z/. Sometimes these consonants are backed to velar place of articulation.

Soft palate

Is there a bifid uvula or lucent zone? These may indicate misalignment of the palate muscles. Is there a fistula? This would be unusual in the soft palate, but may result in nasal emission or hypernasality.

Tongue

Check the tongue mobility, although this is unlikely to be a cleft-related problem *per se*, even if there is incorrect tongue placement for some consonant sounds.

Tonsils

If these are very large they may interfere with palate movement. In addition they may occasionally reduce intra-oral pressure, resulting in the classic 'hot potato' voice quality.

Consideration of influencing factors

When planning therapy it is important to identify any factors that may influence the effectiveness and outcome of the therapy programme. Such factors include structural anomalies, hearing impairment, motivation, age, cognitive level, support available from a parent, carer or other appropriate person and logistical factors.

Structural anomalies

The presence of structural anomalies should not preclude therapy. Even when velopharyngeal dysfunction is suspected or confirmed, therapy should continue in order to facilitate normal patterns of articulation (Le Blanc, 1996; Russell & Harding, 2001). In fact, progress with articulation therapy is often part of the decision-making process when velopharyngeal surgery is being considered. However, as Sell and Grunwell (2001) discuss, the timing of velopharyngeal surgery in relation to therapy is a difficult and controversial area.

Reports have indicated that therapy prior to surgery facilitates the development of normal articulatory patterns, confirms the diagnosis and need for surgery, may result in less obstructive velopharyngeal surgery and can produce more positive post-operative results (Golding-Kushner, 1995; Le Blanc, 1996; Russell, 1997). However, it has also been argued that providing a client with a more efficient velopharyngeal mechanism can facilitate speech therapy (Albery et al, 1986; McWilliams et al, 1990; Van Demark & Hardin, 1990). Sell and Grunwell (2001) comment that surgical timing may in part be determined by the surgical approach and recommend a period of diagnostic articulation therapy, together with careful documentation of articulation change.

Dental and occlusal anomalies, and residual clefts or fistulae, may also impose articulatory constraints and these will need to be taken into account in therapy. However, as Grundy and Harding (1995) point out 'it is possible for different articulatory gestures to produce a sound which is perceptually the same'. Therapy may, therefore, involve exploring alternative or adaptive ways to produce the target consonant.

Hearing impairment

As Lennox (2001) describes, 'the association between cleft palate and ear disease is well established'. There is a high incidence of otitis media caused by Eustachian tube malfunction. This results in a conductive hearing loss, which may fluctuate and can seriously affect auditory skills and communication development (Bamford & Saunders, 1990). Although the hearing abilities of children with cleft palate will be monitored regularly as part of their care pathway, there may be times when therapy is being implemented and the child is also suffering from a hearing loss. The therapist needs to be aware of this possibility and take it into account in therapy sessions ensuring that the child can hear sufficiently for specific tasks. Sitting opposite the child during activities can be particularly helpful.

Motivation

Changing speech patterns can be difficult for clients and requires attention, concentration and a commitment to regular practice.

Motivating children

Young children can easily be motivated with simple rewards of stickers or games but motivating older children can be more challenging. However, therapy can be facilitated if specific motivating goals are identified. There needs to be discussion between the therapist, the parent or carer and the child, with ground rules being clearly established and understood by all parties (Russell & Sell, 1998). The importance of parental involvement in identifying the reward and monitoring the points system established to achieve it is obviously essential. The parent must also be prepared to withhold the reward until the points have genuinely been earned so the goal must be realistic. A reward system is not effective in all cases and sometimes alternative strategies need to be adopted. Russell and Sell (1998) describe a case where a reward system could not be identified and home practice was not carried out. With the help of the child's school, a sympathetic sixth former was identified to help the child on a regular basis.

Motivating adults

Adult clients also need to be highly motivated. They must be prepared to invest considerable time and effort in learning and maintaining new articulatory gestures while inhibiting habitual patterns. It is possible for the older client to achieve quite significant and positive changes. However, it may be necessary to explore in some depth psychological aspects of therapy related to self-image, the expectations of friends and family, and the intrinsic desire of the individual to change.

Age and cognitive level

Different therapy approaches and techniques are needed according to the age and cognitive level of the client. When early intervention is needed, home programmes are usually the most appropriate method of provision. Parents are taught how to facilitate and reinforce appropriate patterns in babble and first words. Therapy for children from about 18 months to three years of age involves a combination of the indirect approach used for younger children and more direct articulation therapy (Russell & Harding, 2001).

Support available

Support for children

Parental support, as illustrated above with regard to reward systems, is particularly important for children, who may be unconcerned about their speech production. In addition it is often appropriate and helpful to involve other family members and older siblings.

Other sources of support may also need to be sought, especially in situations where it is difficult for this to be provided by the immediate family. Nursery and school staff are often valuable contributors to the therapy programme. Although it may be time-consuming for the therapist to liaise with these sources of support this expenditure is outweighed by the benefits to the child: in the long term, their involvement may well shorten the duration of the therapy programme.

It is, however, essential that the therapist ensures that each person working with the child understands and carries out tasks in the right way. Feedback to the child must be accurate so that habitual errors are not reinforced. It is all too easy to unwittingly reinforce cleft type consonant errors; for example, accepting /k/ as correct when the target is /t/, or glottal reinforcement accompanying attempts to produce plosive consonants.

Support for adult clients

Adult clients are also helped by having someone to listen to and monitor their speech practice. When there is no one available, using video or audio recorders to provide feedback can be very effective (Russell & Sell, 1998).

Logistical factors

Logistical factors are related to support and contribute to the decisions regarding who is going to carry out the therapy, when, where and how often. Dodd (1995) discusses the 'practicalities of the provision of therapy' and illustrates how the benefits to be gained from attending formal therapy sessions may be outweighed by the disadvantages. In other words, it may be difficult for the client to attend because of transport difficulties, parents' (or in the case of adults, their own) working commitments, other demands on time and conflicting priorities.

It is evident from the literature and clinical experience that children with cleft palate respond best to focused, intensive therapy (Golding-Kushner, 1995; Hoch *et al*, 1986; Le Blanc, 1996). However, logistical factors may mean that there has to be a compromise with regard to the frequency of therapy sessions. Progress can still be made provided that the therapy programme is appropriate and that there is consistent daily follow-up. Different models of provision, ranging from home- and school-based programmes to regular intensive therapy, should be considered.

There may be times when the therapist decides that the influencing factors cannot be overcome. Following discussion with parents, carers and/or the client it may be necessary to recommend that therapy is deferred for a while. This can occur in cases where motivation is a problem, where surgical treatment is planned or when orthodontic treatment is taking place.

It is important that there is close liaison between the therapist on the cleft palate team and the local therapist about any issues associated with the implementation of the therapy programme. This is vital when a decision to defer therapy may be made. In order to plan for effective therapy there needs to be close collaboration between the two therapists. A contribution from both is required so that the full picture with regard to influencing factors is obtained. This helps to clarify situations, for example, where the cleft team therapist is recommending further therapy but the local therapist is becoming increasingly disillusioned as the child is not progressing with weekly sessions.

If deferment of therapy is indicated, it is important that the client is reviewed within a specific time frame. In the case of older clients, however, it may be appropriate to give them the responsibility of contacting the therapist in order to initiate a review or further therapy.

Intervention

Selection of therapy model

The age of the child and the results of the assessment will indicate whether direct or indirect intervention by the speech and language therapist is required.

Indirect intervention

Indirect intervention involves the parents carrying out with the child, specific activities which have been suggested by the therapist. This is particularly appropriate for babies and younger children, and includes input modelling and other techniques (see Chapter 2). The advantage of such an approach is that activities can be carried out on a regular basis as part of the child's daily routine. Therapy thus becomes a more natural process and actively involves the parents from the start.

Direct intervention

Direct therapy is when the therapist works with the child and the parents on an individual basis. In some cases a combination of both direct and indirect intervention may be required and it is, of course, essential that there is daily home practice between therapy sessions.

Formulation of the therapy programme

Frequency

With regard to frequency of therapy, as described above, the literature recommends intensive therapy, that is, between three and five times a week. However, positive changes can be achieved with weekly or less frequent sessions provided that therapy is correctly targeted, motivation is in place and there is appropriate daily home practice and support. As Russell and Sell (1998) discuss, therapy usually needs to continue for longer than the six- to eight-week block model. Many of the clients in the *GOS-CLAPA Therapy Project* (Russell & Sell, 1998) were only just beginning to achieve changes at this stage of their treatment and to stop then would have meant that these changes would not have been maintained. Intervention would, therefore, have been ineffective. In fact, this is what had happened to many of these clients before with their previous therapy (Russell & Sell, 1998). It is also one of the reasons that children with cleft palate stay on the caseloads of community therapists for unacceptably long periods of time without progressing.

Focusing on the needs of the child

Lack of progress may also occur when therapy is not accurately focused on the needs of the individual child; for example, if the child is placed in a phonology group when the focus of therapy should be the elicitation and production of specific consonants. It is, however, appropriate to include children with cleft palate in groups with non-cleft palate children, provided that the needs of the children in the group are similar. When there are not enough children with comparable therapy requirements, it may be effective to include just two or three together in therapy sessions.

Younger children with cleft palate who evidence delay in communication development will, of course, benefit from being included in early language groups and given similar opportunities. It is, however, beneficial to them and to the other children in the group if activities include some copying and sound-making activities aimed at promoting phonetic development. It should be remembered that early sound development precedes and is directly related to language development (Stark, 1986).

For children who have completed phonological development (that is, those of five years or older), individual therapy is most often appropriate, with group therapy being used to aid motivation and generalisation of consonants. Intensive group therapy for these older children is described by Albery and Enderby (1984), who used intensive articulation therapy, and Grunwell and Dive (1988), who used a combined articulation and phonological approach. Group therapy can be particularly effective for children presenting with active nasal fricatives (see Chapter 5).

Summary

In summary, the therapy process involves:

- assessment
- consideration of influencing factors
- intervention:
  - selection of therapy model
  - formulation of therapy programme
  - implementation of programme using appropriate therapy techniques and rewards, as described in the remainder of this book.

Pre-Speech and Early Speech Development

Articulation in children aged two years and under

The effects of early intervention

What do we mean by early intervention, and is it effective in preventing or changing cleft-type characteristics? If by 'early' we mean under two years of age, then the jury is still out on whether intervention improves speech outcome by, say, the age of four. To date there have been no large-scale studies proving that active intervention in the very early period is helpful; therefore some may argue that it is not justified on the grounds of cost to the National Health Service and burden to the parents. However, proponents of early intervention (Russell & Harding, 2001, Golding-Kushner, 2001) argue that as therapists we must intervene as soon as we identify cleft-type characteristics and work with parents to remediate them.

Characteristics of pre-speech and early speech development

So, what do we know about this early period in articulatory terms? Research has confirmed the deviant nature of pre-speech development in children with cleft palate (Russell & Grunwell, 1993). Unsurprisingly, pre-operative vocalisations are characterised by deviant and restricted sound development, a lack of labial and lingual plosives and a dominance of glottal and pharyngeal articulations. This phonetic deviance is undoubtedly physically based and results from the structural inadequacy of the intra-oral mechanism.

Following palatoplasty, when there is an improved intra-oral mechanism, children's vocalisations progress towards more normal patterns but phonetic deviance characteristic of the cleft palate condition persists for many children. At about two months post-palatoplasty, Russell and Grunwell (1993) report an increase in lingual articulations, fewer glottal and pharyngeal articulations and an increased occurrence of plosives. There is still a lack of labial and lingual plosives.

By 18 months of age, most children demonstrate further development of lingual plosives and fricatives, but with continued evidence of deviant and restricted sound development. Moreover, at this age individual differences indicate that some children are at risk for speech problems. These phonetic characteristics continue to be present in the early word stage, revealing a relationship between the phonetic and phonological development of these children. The children resolve their deviant speech patterns at different stages and to different extents. It is very important to identify the presence of velopharyngeal insufficiency as soon as possible because this has such a negative influence on phonetic development.

Activities

The activities that follow are intended for use with babies and toddlers when there is evidence of delayed or deviant phonetic development, in particular, delayed development of plosive consonants. The activities may need some adaptation according to the needs of the child, but can be commenced during the pre-speech stage of development and well before 18 months. These ideas would usually be incorporated into a programme to be carried out by the parents at home. For an example of a home programme that may be carried out by parents, and which can be photocopied, please see Appendix 1. It is important that the therapist goes through the programme in detail with the parents and demonstrates the activities. It must be emphasised that all activities, and in particular output activities, should be relaxed and effortless for the child in order to try and avoid the development of abnormal compensatory patterns, for example glottal productions resulting from excess effort.

Philosophy

The overall philosophy of the activities is based on what the child is doing naturally, to reinforce and encourage appropriate development. Parents and carers are taught how to model consonants in participative babble. The more children see, hear and feel particular sounds that are repeatedly modelled in specific ways, the more likely they are to produce similar sounds themselves (Stoel-Gammon, 1992). As Russell and Harding (2001) discuss, such an approach enables the acquisition of new sounds to be completely effortless for the child. They also comment that parents should be advised to interpret babbled utterances as potentially meaningful in order to encourage vocal output. The therapist should discuss with the parents how the activities can be incorporated into the child's daily routine so that advantage can be taken of naturally occurring opportunities. Many of the suggestions are for the type of activities that people routinely engage in with young children. It should be explained to the parents that there is a need to continue with such activities, especially when the child is not yet able to produce the desired response. It may be appropriate to involve others, for example older siblings and grandparents, with the therapy programme.

Review

It is important for the therapist to review progress regularly, preferably at least at monthly intervals. It may be appropriate to combine direct therapy sessions (when the therapist interacts with the child) with indirect therapy (a programme of activities to be carried out at home). Russell and Harding (2001) point out that some parents need to have repeated demonstrations of modelling techniques before they are confident to apply them. Videotapes of modelled activities are effective in helping parents to carry out the programme and extend the therapeutic experience into the home. Some children are already aware of their difficulties and may be reluctant to attempt production tasks such as imitation of consonants. These activities, therefore, need to be introduced in a subtle manner through modelling activities within games and normal daily routines. At some stages during input-modelling, for example, a vocal response from the child may not be expected (Harding-Bell & Bryan, 2003). This must all be discussed in detail with the parents.

Aims

The activities that follow aim to:

- encourage a wider range of speech-like vocalisations and for children to 'experiment' with their articulators in **babble and input modelling sessions**
- encourage gross motor and articulatory **imitation**
- promote the development of **listening skills**
- increase **auditory discrimination** and awareness
- increase oral sensitivity and awareness
- encourage oral direction of airstream.

There may be other aims relating to language development, as required.

Babble and input modelling sessions

Participative babble sessions

Good times for engaging in these sessions may be when changing the child, at the beginning or end of the day, at bathtime or whenever the child seems particularly communicative. Start with strings of sounds that the child can easily achieve, for example /lala, wəwə, məmə, nana/, and move on to other easy ones. Vary the vowel sounds and also the volume and intonation patterns. During this activity, encourage the child to feel your face and lips, and his own. When appropriate, for example at bathtime, babble on or near different parts of the child's body (such as arms, hands, back, abdomen, tummy, cheeks). Encourage the child to reciprocate in a similar manner.

Once some success is achieved, and the child is participating in and enjoying these sessions, different sounds can be introduced alongside those that the child can achieve. Remember to use 'desirable', that is, 'normal' speech-like consonant and vowel sounds. Explain this to parents and show them how to reinforce 'normal' sounds and to ignore 'undesirable' sounds, such as glottal and pharyngeal productions.

Using games to model pitch and intonation

When swinging the child or playing 'horse' games on your lap, vary your pitch and intonation. For example, say 'up' with a rising inflection and 'down' with a falling inflection, at the appropriate stage in the game. If the child tries to imitate the intonational pattern, repeat the activity several times. With toddlers this can be carried over into other situations, such as going up and down stairs, riding on a seesaw and so on.

Repetitive songs and nursery rhymes

When you sing simple songs and nursery rhymes, encourage the child to join in with the melody and the words as much as he can. 'Round and round the garden' and 'peek-a-boo' games can also be used. Use the pitch of your voice and your inflection to communicate emotions such as joy, anger and surprise. You may need to over-emphasise these at first.

Animal, vehicle and general everyday noises

Use suitable items from the child's toys, pictures and environment to model common sounds and noises, for example a dog, cat, baby, car, train, aeroplane, vacuum cleaner, shower, telephone or kettle. Recordings of some of these sounds with corresponding pictures are available commercially but where possible parents should be encouraged to use everyday opportunities, always associating the same sound with the particular object.

Imitate the sound yourself, using the associated visual and auditory cues to identify what you are doing. Use any opportunity to demonstrate 'desirable' sounds, for example a /ʃ/ sound might be associated with a shower and /t t t/ with a dripping tap. 'Bubble-wobbling' by saying /p/ to make a bubble on a wand move, particularly helps to attract the child's attention (Harding-Bell & Bryan, 2003). Avoid 'abnormal' sounds, such as glottal plosives. Make sure any 'growls' use /r/-type sounds rather than throat noises. If the sounds are associated with items on a regular and consistent basis as part of a game, the child will be encouraged to attempt to copy them.

Imitation

These activities help to encourage the child to copy specific physical movements spontaneously and naturally. It is often easier to start with gross motor activities so that the child learns to appreciate the general enjoyment of copying games. Subsequently, it is easier to move on to more precise copying of tongue and lip movements and sounds. It may help if some of these activities are carried out in front of a mirror (preferably a full length mirror for the gross motor activities).

Gross motor imitation

Encourage the child to copy whole body movements, such as clapping, dancing, jumping and banging or tapping on a table or drum. Make the game slightly harder as the child achieves success. Such activities may be incorporated into a 'Simon says' or any type of 'Follow the leader' game. It is helpful to have other children and/or adults joining in with this activity; in fact, you should encourage anything that invites the child to watch and copy. A similar activity is to link the game with everyday actions in the manner of a song 'This is the way we ...' (brush our hair, clean our teeth, wash our face, wave goodbye and so on).

Move on to gross motor movements of the face, such as smiling, frowning, exaggerated yawning and blinking. Emphasise and encourage the child to copy facial expressions associated with happy/sad, a nasty smell, surprise (associated with 'peek-a-boo' game) and other suitable expressions. From this activity you can move on to imitation of tongue and lip movements.

Imitation of tongue and lip movements

Encourage the child to copy specific lip shapes, associating the desired shape/sound with a specific object and action; for example /o/, a rounded lip shape, with a fish; pursed lips and /ʃ/ with 'the baby's sleeping; /ee/ lips spread with a clown face. Make exaggerated /oo/ and /ah/ noises with different facial expressions. Make faces in a mirror, including for example, pursed lips with an appropriate sound to indicate 'kissing'.

Imitation of tongue movements starts with protruding the tongue and just putting it in and out of the mouth, then learning to move it from side to side. You can then progress to up (to top lip and towards nose) and down (towards chin) movements. Following this, try for imitation of tongue movements *inside* the mouth, for example putting the tongue up behind the top teeth. It is very useful to use the concept of Mr Tongue as portrayed in the 'Mr Tongue' story (Dudley South PCT). The 'Mighty Mouth' board game is also helpful for imitation activities. For details of both these Resources, see Appendix 4.

Listening skills

Sounds in the environment

Identify sounds in the environment and play 'What can we hear?' Use sounds like those suggested above in the babbling and imitation games. In fact, the listening and imitation activities will probably be carried out simultaneously.

Listening to recordings

Use recordings of familiar tunes, noises and voices. Turn the volume very low and ask the child to help you to identify the tune.

Following whispered instructions

Play games in which the child has to follow whispered instructions. Encourage the child and others playing the games (such as siblings) to take a turn at being the instructor.

Listening for the hidden object

Use toys and objects that make a noise, such as a music box, clock, egg timer or radio. Take turns in hiding the object in different places and find it by listening for the sound it makes.

Auditory discrimination

Identifying different sound makers

Use different sound makers, such as a whistle, bell or rattle. A variety of the child's own toys can be used, together with some household items (for example, a spoon in a cup). Show the parents how to teach the child to identify each object by the noise it makes: first, by letting the child see the objects and later by hiding them behind a 'screen'.

What's in the box?

Suggest that the parents collect a number of identical containers (for example, margarine tubs with lids) and fill them with items that will make a noise when the tub is shaken. The child is required to identify the item in the tub by the noise it makes (for example, toy bricks versus sand) or to match two tubs with identical contents. Very different sounds can be used to start with, but as the child succeeds, more similar sounds can be used.

Which picture?

Use a set of different pictures. The child selects the one you say. Gradually reduce the volume of your voice during this activity. In a more advanced version of the same game, the child selects a picture from a choice of minimal pair words, such as *cat, hat, bat*. The number of pictures to choose from will vary from about three to eight, depending on the age and ability of the child.

Oral direction of airstream

It is essential to understand that these activities are aimed at helping children to learn to produce an oral airstream for consonant production. They are definitely *not* exercises to promote palate or velopharyngeal function and it has been clearly shown that they do not work as such (Golding-Kushner, 2001; Sell & Grunwell, 2001). However, some children do need to learn how to direct air through their mouth and from acquiring this ability may subsequently be able produce specific consonants. For example, /f/ may be developed from gentle direction of air orally with lips close together, leading to a bilabial fricative that can then be modified with dental involvement to become /f/.

Care must be taken with the vocabulary used in these activities in order to avoid any excess effort that may be associated with words such as 'blowing'. It is sometimes better to focus on a task such as the activity below.

Wobble the bubble/Roll the ball

Tell the child, 'Let's make the bubble wobble for as long as we can' (by saying /p p p/) or 'Let's make the (tissue) ball roll over the table'. Parents must understand that the emphasis is on gentle airflow that will subsequently be modified with movements of the lips and tongue. Nose-holding often helps the child to experience oral versus nasal airflow. Often the completeness of constriction of the nose can be gradually lessened so that eventually just a finger touching the nose serves to remind the child about using an oral airstream.

Feel the air

When first eliciting an oral airstream, let the child 'feel the air' when you direct it gently from your mouth onto his hand or against very lightweight objects such as feathers and pieces of tissue.

Make it cooler!

Gently use an oral airstream to cool hot food in a real or pretend situation. Encourage the child to copy you in a relaxed and gentle manner.

When success is achieved, start to modify the airstream using your lips and tongue, as in the 'bubble-wobbling' activity described above.

Blowing bubbles through a straw

In some games, a straw or piece of plastic tubing may be used. Holding the straw centrally in the mouth and gently 'blowing' bubbles in water can help in the achievement of a central airstream and forward tongue position for the eventual production of /s/.

Developing a Speech Sound System

Moving from pre-speech to speech

The activities in this chapter provide a link between the pre-speech activities described in Chapter 2 and the more specific articulation programme described in Chapter 4.

Activities

Aims

The broad aims of these activities are much the same as for the pre-speech section, but more 'speech' work is gradually introduced. The activities aim to:

- encourage the child to use consonants correctly and to use them more often and in different word positions
- encourage the child's awareness of different speech sounds and to improve listening and discrimination skills
- encourage the child to experiment with his articulators in order to learn how to produce new consonants
- produce consonants with correct articulatory placement (and, if possible, the appropriate manner of articulation, for example plosive or fricative).

Auditory discrimination

Using picture cards

Associate consonants and vowels with specific pictures, for example /s/ with a snake. Depending on the needs and age of the child, the therapist will select the most appropriate sound/picture association system. There is a choice of published systems including the Nuffield Centre Dyspraxia Programme and Mr Big Mouth (see Appendix 4).

Make cards using the chosen system and introduce some of the sounds to the child. Start with three or four very different sounds (for example /m/, /g/ and /l/), building up to more and increasing the difficulty (using similar sounds, for example a range of fricatives) when the child is achieving success.

Picture card games

With the three or four selected sounds, play games in which the child is required to find the picture of the sound he hears. When the child identifies the sound correctly he achieves a 'reward'. For example:

- the child 'wins' pieces to put in a jigsaw or form board
- the child puts a brick on the correct picture and builds towers
- the child pushes a toy car to the correct picture
- the child jumps on the correct picture
- the child 'wins' an item such as a marble or small car which is used in play at the end of the activity
- Stickers or stars are put next to the appropriate picture.

Making the task more difficult

When the child is achieving 100 per cent success with sounds in isolation (consonants and vowels, as required) move on to listening for consonant sounds in consonant + vowel (CV) and vowel + consonant (VC) syllables and words.

It is important to achieve success at each stage before gradually making the task more difficult, as described above. When the child has become proficient at identifying the required sound or sounds in CV and VC words, move on to simple CVC and then CVCV words. The ultimate objective is for the child to be able to recognise different consonants in all word positions; that is, word initially (WI), within word (WW) and word finally (WF). For most children it is easier to start with WI position, but some may respond better to hearing consonants in WF position. Listening for WW consonants often comes much later in the programme.

From babble to speech sound production

From the babble sessions, imitation games and the child's spontaneous production attempts, the therapist will be able to identify which sounds the child can produce. Another advantage of the discrimination games described above is that many children will spontaneously start to copy the consonants and vowels. This can be taken further through imitation games in which the child is encouraged to produce different speech sounds for a reward.

Target selection

When choosing which consonant sounds to work on, it is important for the therapist to be guided by the child's ability and the overall aims of the therapy programme. For example, the therapist may want to focus on labial or front of tongue sounds. It is often appropriate to ignore developmental guidelines when working with this population. Some children find it easier to produce fricatives than plosives at first. Similarly, voiceless consonants may be easier than voiced. This is particularly applicable when velopharyngeal dysfunction is suspected. Fricative and voiceless sounds are likely to be easier for the child to produce, and by focusing on these it may be possible to prevent the development of abnormal patterns such as glottal and pharyngeal articulations.

It is advisable at first to concentrate on a range of different consonants, including those that the child *does* produce as well as those he *does not*. Vowels should also be included. In this way, some real success is built into the task, which does not focus specifically on any one consonant. This activity should be introduced to the parents or carers very carefully and monitored closely by the therapist to ensure that the child is not put under pressure. It is important to stress to the parents that the child is not necessarily expected to succeed in imitating all the consonants. The aim is to encourage and reinforce his attempts at imitating the correct articulatory placement rather than the results *per se*, particularly when there may be velopharyngeal dysfunction. In addition, the child is being encouraged to experiment with his articulators in order to 'discover' new sounds that he can produce.

When there has been some success with elicitation of a target consonant the therapist may decide to focus particularly on that consonant in order to stabilise its production (see 'Drill' below). Even when doing this, however, it is still a good idea to include some 'sound experimentation' within the therapy session. Experienced therapists will be aware of occasions when children suddenly demonstrate their ability to produce a different consonant. This may then result in new and different aims as the therapist takes advantage of the child's achievement.

Using the same sound/picture association as for the auditory discrimination activities described above (and often in conjunction with those activities) games can be devised in which the child is required to attempt to copy and produce a specific sound for a reward. At first, any attempt should be rewarded; as the child becomes more confident in participating in the activity, the therapist may request more accuracy. Some nose holding may be used as an aid to achieving oral consonants and can help the child to experience the appropriate sensation. The 'rewards' may be similar to those in the activities described above for auditory discrimination. Most children enjoy 'earning' a ball to put on a stick, a star to stick on, a picture to colour and other similar rewards.

Drill

When a new consonant has been successfully achieved it needs to be practised over and over again; that is, drilled until it is always produced correctly. As Golding-Kushner (1995) comments, 'drill is often regarded as an uninteresting procedure of last resort' but 'with motivating stimuli and reinforcement materials, an upbeat clinician attitude and fast pace, it is highly effective'. Drill is an extension of the production games described above. It is used to consolidate production of a sound in isolation and then in CV, VC and consonant sequences. The Nuffield Centre Dyspraxia Programme provides some useful pictorial activities that require the child to repeatedly produce the same consonant or sequences of consonants. Children usually enjoy receiving a sticker as their reward for this activity.

Putting sounds together

When the child is confidently and consistently producing different vowels and consonants in the games described above, move towards producing a sequence of two sounds. The combinations may be consonant + consonant (CC), vowel + vowel (VV), CV or VC. The exercises that form part of the Nuffield Centre Dyspraxia Programme and require the child to repeatedly produce a sequence of two or three consonants (for example, /p, k, p, k, p, k/) are particularly useful for this activity. Similar sequencing games can be constructed using different sound/picture association systems and these will help the child to maintain production of the target consonant.

At this stage two sounds can be combined to form meaningful words. However, the therapist needs to be aware of the dangers of moving on too quickly. It is important to make sure that a production is stable before attempting it in words because of the dangers of therapy-induced errors, such as double articulation and glottal reinforcement. The sequencing activities described above can help to avoid these, as can hand stroking.

Hand stroking

It can sometimes be difficult to teach the child how to achieve a smooth transition between the components of CV and VC syllables. One method of doing this is to use hand stroking (Harding-Bell & Bryan, 2003; Jeremy, personal communication). Hands are usually palm down and it can be useful to draw round the hand so that there is also a pictorial representation. The centre of the hand represents the target consonant and the tip of each finger and the thumb represent vowels. Gently stroke from the centre to the end of each digit while demonstrating smooth transition from consonant to vowel, for example, /fff ... ee/ or /p ... aa/. At first the child may just listen and watch, and he can then be encouraged to join in. Children tend to like the sensation of their hand being stroked and this activity focuses their attention so that often even the liveliest child becomes still. Stroking can start from the tips of the fingers to the centre of the hand for VC syllables.

Case example

Session plan for Zoë

This is a real example that was used with a two-and-a-half year old girl, Zoë. The overall aims of the session are those listed above, with specific targets in mind. The activities often cover more than one aim. Zoë's mother observes all the sessions, which are approximately one hour long. At the beginning of therapy Zoë was communicating using vowels and intonation with very few consonants. However, in the first session she was stimulable for /p/ as well as nasals and approximants. Table 1 shows Zoë's fourth therapy session.

TABLE 1 Session plan for Zoë, aged two years and six months

Plan	Activity	Materials
Listening / Discrimination of /p k j m w/ in isolation.	a revise picture / sound association while getting pictures out. b Zoë to put 'figure' on sound she hears therapist say. Continue until three figures on each sound.	Sound pictures on cards (from *Nuffield Dyspraxia Programme*). People figures.
General sound imitation task. Imitation of new sound.	a Imitation of /p b m n k f/ b Imitation of new sound /f/ c Try to elicit other consonants, for example /l/ and dental /t/ and /d/	Reward each production with ball to put on stick or item for game to play at end of activity (for example, sword from 'Pop up Pirate').
Repeated consonant sequences.	a /w/ /m/ b /w/ /j/ c /p/ /k/ Zoë puts her finger on each sound as she says it.	'Ladders' from *Nuffield Dyspraxia Programme*.
Production of CVCV words, for example, *mummy, nanny, pepper, poppy, car key.*	Hide pictures around the room for Zoë to find and identify.	CVCV pictures from *Nuffield Dyspraxia Programme*.
Homework discussion Zoë's mother already has the Mr Tongue story (see Appendix 4) and she has put the sound pictures onto cards.	**Play activity for Zoë.** I ask her mother to make sure Zoë can find the picture when she hears the sound and to play around with consonant production using the cards, ladders and CVCV words.	*Nuffield Dyspraxia Programme* ladders and CVCV words.

Structuring Articulation Programmes

A staged and structured approach to changing cleft-type characteristics is recommended. This approach is suitable for children of three years plus, depending on level of co-operation.

Pre-production strategies

Before commencing a programme such as this it is assumed that a comprehensive assessment of a child's consonant system has been made and consonants for remediation identified.

Auditory discrimination and recognition should be checked but it is not usually necessary to spend as much time on this pre-production as a therapist would, for example, for a purely phonological difficulty. It is recommended that pictures of minimal pairs are used for testing and remediating auditory discrimination and recognition.

Selecting target consonants

From the consonants needing remediation in the child's system, select first those which give visual cues, for example /p, f, t/. Voiceless consonants seem to be easier to produce as a 'new' sound than voiced so start with voiceless.

Keep phonological development in mind so affricates and clusters can usually be left until last.

The articulation programme

The following five stages are recommended for an effective articulation programme (Morley, 1970; Golding-Kushner, 2001).

1 Eliciting a target consonant in isolation
2 Eliciting VC and CV combinations
3 Eliciting single words
4 Eliciting short sentences
5 Generalisation.

The most difficult stages tend to be the first and last.

Eliciting a target consonant in isolation

Always test imitation of a target consonant first. If this is not successful, the techniques described in Table 2 can be tried. Plosives, fricatives and affricates only are included, these being the most common consonants needing remediation.

Golding-Kushner (2001) recommends the use of a sustained /h/ to break a glottal pattern for any oral consonant. To use /h/ as a facilitator, easy oral airflow for /h/ should be sustained and the appropriate oral movements may then be overlaid to produce the other sounds.

At this level, helpful publications are the *Black Sheep Consonant Worksheets*, *Nuffield Centre Dyspraxia Programme* pictures and *Jolly Phonics* (see Jolly Learning, Appendix 4). An example from the Black Sheep series is reproduced in Figure 1 on page 32.

TABLE 2 Consonant elicitation techniques

Consonant	Technique
/p/	A gentle /p/ sound can be introduced in the middle of a gentle blow or sustained /h/. Use a paper tissue or paper apples on a tree so the 'wind' blows the objects when an oral /p/ is produced.
/b/	Use nasal /m/ as a facilitator. Ask the child to say /maː/ a few times, then use nose-holding for the final /maː/, which will then sound like /baː/. Practise with nose-holding until /baː/ can be produced without. Sometimes simply describing /b/ as a noisy /p/ and feeling the vibration from the larynx will work.
/t/	This is an important consonant to obtain as it can lead to other alveolar or palato-alveolar consonants. Use /h/ as a facilitator and try gentle 'tongue-tapping' making a non-aspirated /t/. Try a labiodental or labiolingual /t/ and gradually move it back to behind the teeth.
/d/	Use nasal /n/ as a facilitator as /m/ can be a facilitator for /b/ (see above). Again, sometimes just describing /d/ as a noisy /t/ can work, or whispering /d/ if /t/ can be produced correctly and then gradually introducing voicing.
/k/ and /g/	Hold the front of the tongue down with a tongue depressor while asking the child to lift up the back of the tongue to make a /k/, shaping a gentle cough. If a nasal plosive, for example /ŋ/, is possible then ask the child to repeat /iŋgi/ producing /ŋg/ in the medial position. When the nose is held a /g/ will be produced. /g/ is usually easier to obtain than /k/, whereas for other sounds the voiceless ones are easier. Once /g/ is correct then a 'whispered' /g/ will produce a /k/.
/f/	Visual feedback using a mirror may be helpful, or feeling the airstream on the back of the hand. A picture of a rabbit with protruding teeth (see Figure 1) is helpful too.
/v/	Usually follows easily from /f/. A 'buzzing' /f/ or noisy /f/.
/θ/	Easy to imitate using a mirror. Once obtained it may be used as a springboard for /s/.
/s/	If /t/ can be produced /s/ is most often obtained from a prolonged /t/, making it into a fricative sound /tsssss/. Alternatively, if /θ/ is possible then moving the tongue behind the teeth while still trying to say /θ/ can work. Occasionally /s/ may be obtained from /ʃ/ by asking the child to spread the lips and move the tongue slightly forward.
/z/	A noisy /s/, feeling the vibration from the larynx and buzz of the tongue tip.
/ʃ/	Usually easier to obtain after /s/. Produce /s/ with lips rounded and place tongue further back.
/ʒ/	Noisy /ʃ/. Feel the vibration of the larynx.
/tʃ/	If /ʃ/ is correct then t + ʃ as in words such as *catch* or *match*. Practising t + j together can also facilitate /tʃ/. Younger children can be asked to make a 'sneezing' sound.
/dʒ/	A noisy /tʃ/ or separating d + j and bringing them gradually closer together.

FIGURE 1 Ferdy Rabbit

Make the 'rabbit' sound.

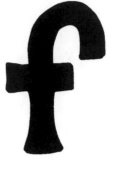

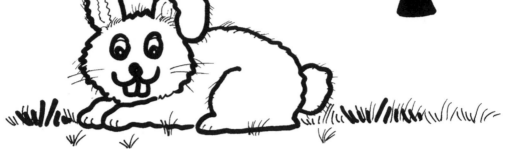

Ferdy Rabbit shows his big teeth when he says this sound!
You show YOUR teeth...

... and BLOW... to make this sound.

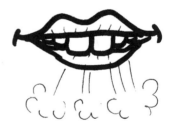

These fish have funny names. Show your teeth when you say their names. Colour them in!

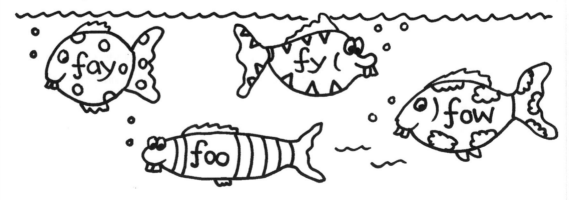

Eliciting VC and CV combinations

Once a target consonant is elicited correctly and is stable, a period of practice at VC and CV level is helpful before moving on to single words. Usually the consonant in final position is easier than that in initial, so try the final position consonant first (Figure 2).

FIGURE 2 Mr Balloon-man

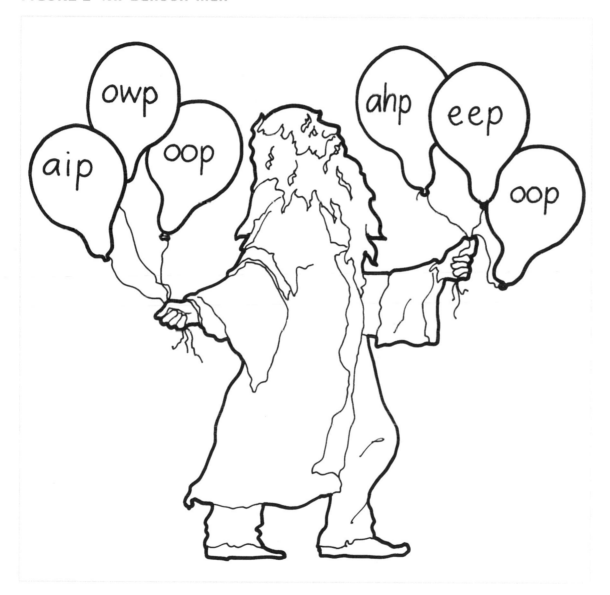

In initial position it may be difficult to integrate the consonant with the vowel and for a short period the therapist can place /h/ between the two, which can then easily be phased out (/p-hi/ or /t-ha:/). Many children can integrate the initial consonant easily with the vowel. Young children may enjoy colouring in an apple on the apple tree as below every time the correct combination is produced (see Figure 3).

FIGURE 3 Apple tree

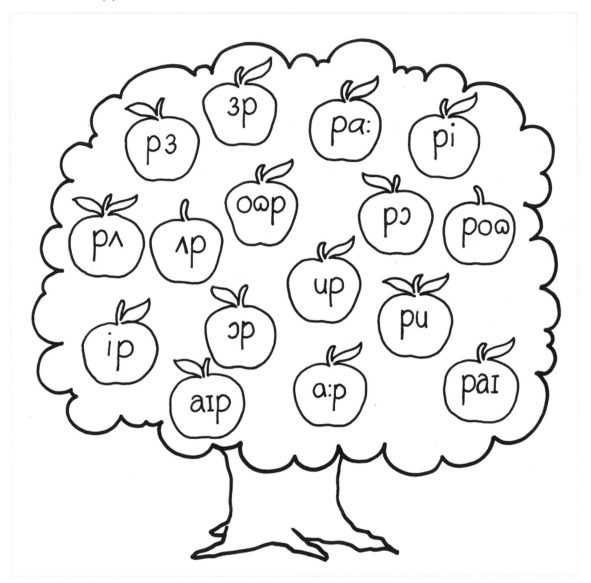

Eliciting single words

For children

For children, illustrate single words with familiar pictures. We recommend the Black Sheep Press consonant worksheets (see Figure 4 and the details in Appendix 4) as well as the examples on the following handouts. Children can be asked simply to name each single word picture or the pictures may be cut out and used in games. In addition, the Clapa Thameside games (see Appendix 4) can be used at this stage.

Please turn to page 70 for activities for adults.

FIGURE 4 Example of initial 'f' worksheet

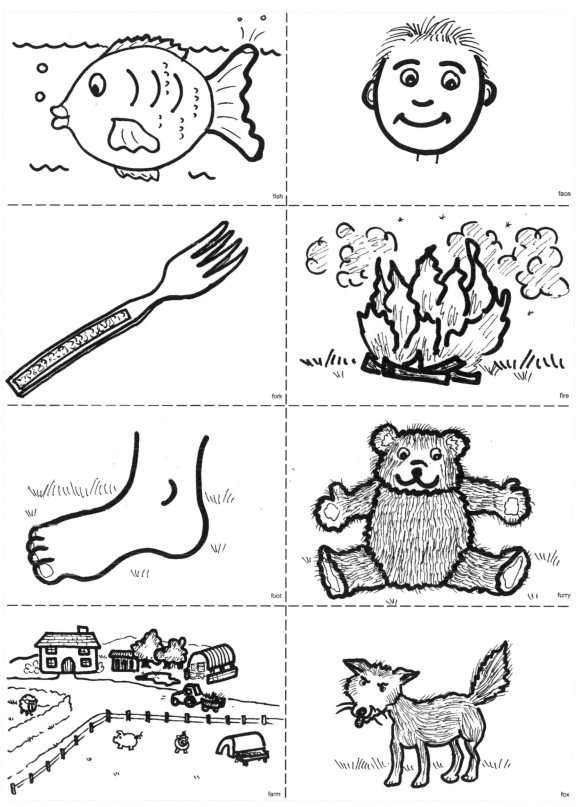

Handout 1 Pictures to elicit articulation of p–

pie	paper
pen	purse
peg	paint

Handout 2 Pictures to elicit articulation of –p

ape	cup
top	tap
soup	rope

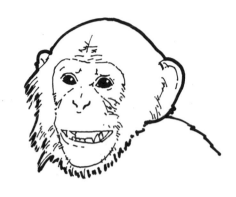

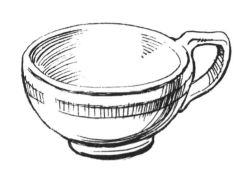

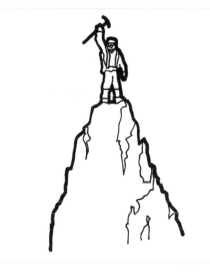

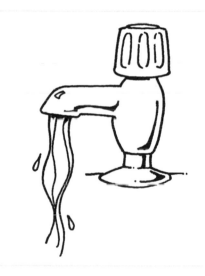

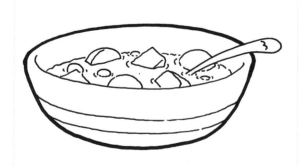

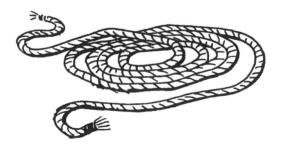

Routledge
Taylor & Francis Group

bat	book
ball	bike
bee	boat

Routledge
Taylor & Francis Group

Handout 4 Pictures to elicit articulation of –b

bib	web
knob	nib
crab	sob

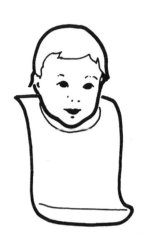

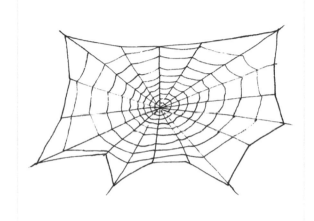

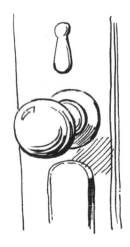

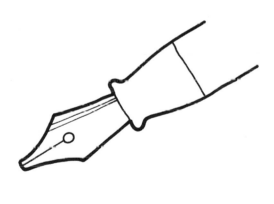

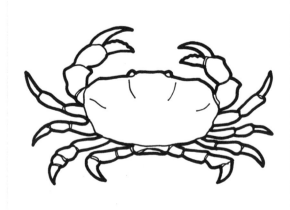

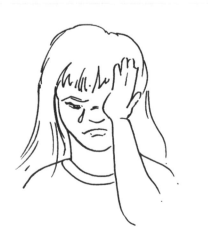

Routledge
Taylor & Francis Group

Handout 5 Pictures to elicit articulation of t–

tea	ten
toe	tin
tail	tie

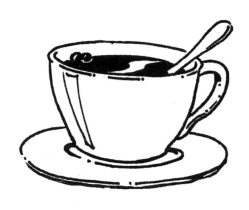

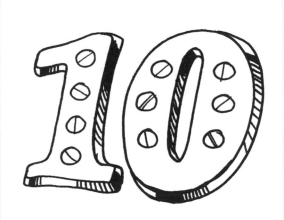

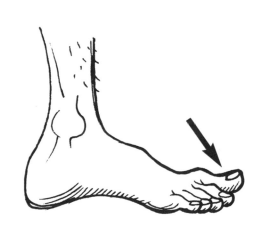

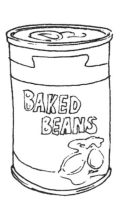

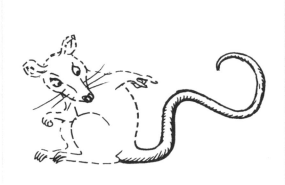

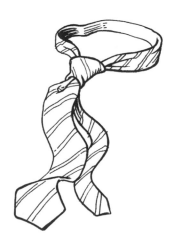

Handout 6 Pictures to elicit articulation of –t

hat	boat
meat	light
boot	eat

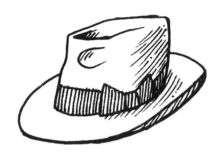

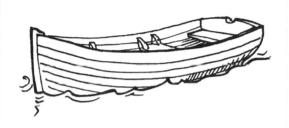

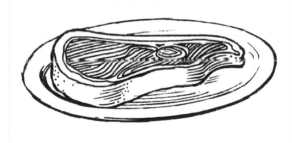

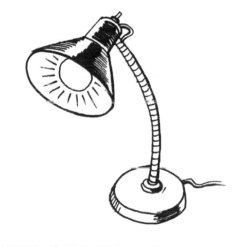

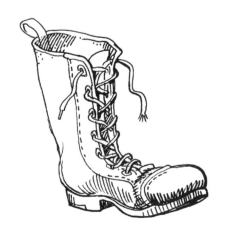

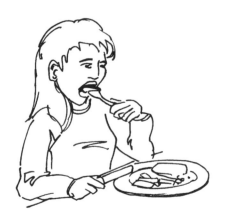

Routledge
Taylor & Francis Group

Handout 7 Pictures to elicit articulation of d–

door	dig
dive	dog
dolphin	duck

Handout 8 Pictures to elicit articulation of –d

road	sword
bead	bed
wood	head

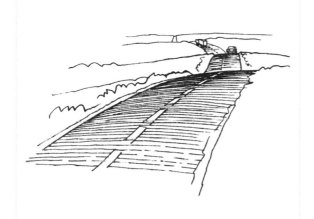

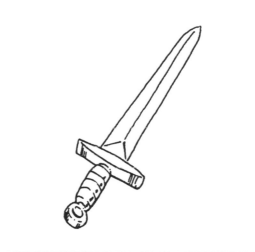

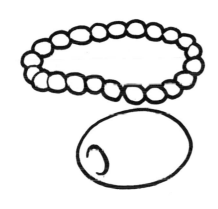

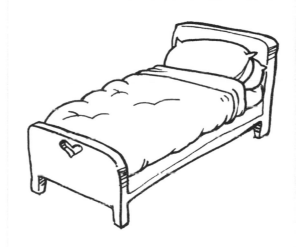

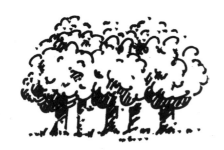

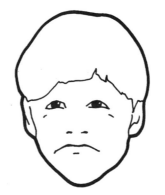

Handout 9 Pictures to elicit articulation of k–

car	cat
cup	cow
cake	key

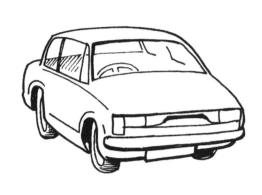
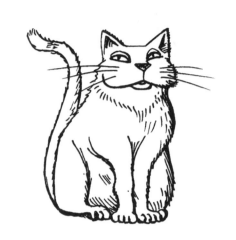
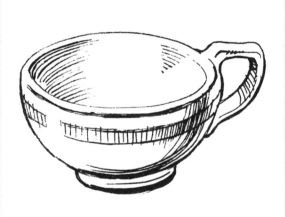
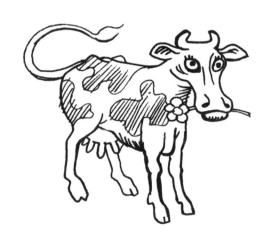
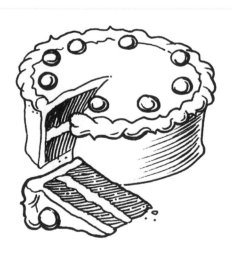
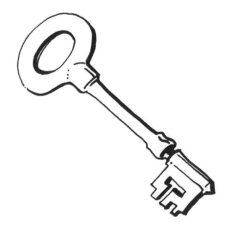

Handout 10 Pictures to elicit articulation of –k

duck	truck
rake	sock
kick	back

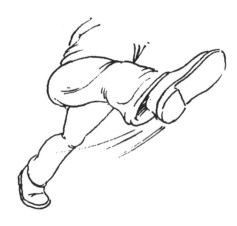
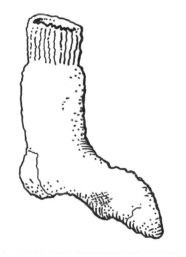
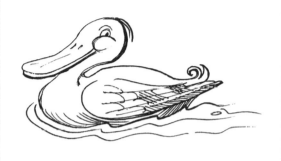
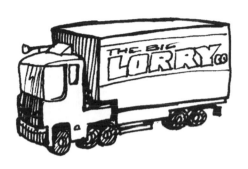
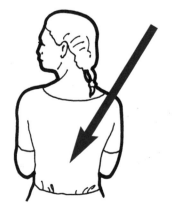
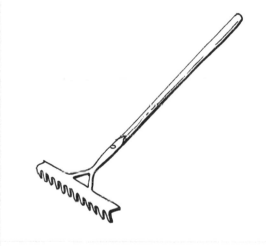

Routledge
Taylor & Francis Group

Handout 11 Pictures to elicit articulation of g–

goal	girl
garden	guitar
gate	garage

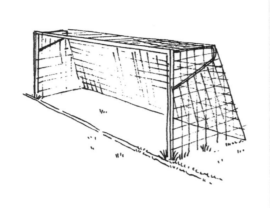 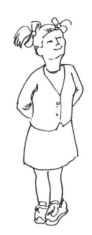

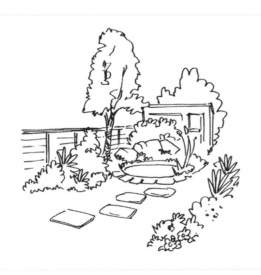 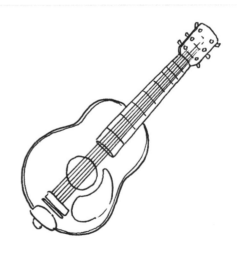

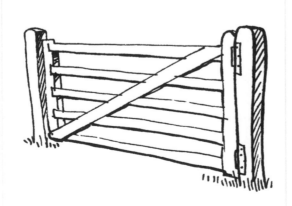 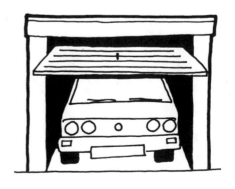

Routledge
Taylor & Francis Group

Handout 12 Pictures to elicit articulation of –g

egg	leg
pig	jug
flag	dog

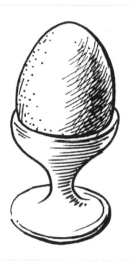

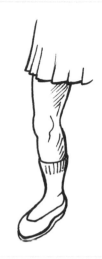

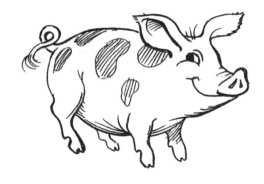

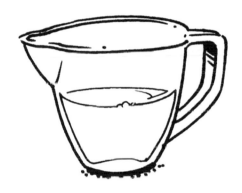

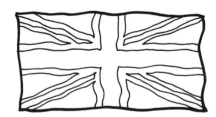

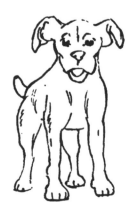

Handout 13 Pictures to elicit articulation of f–

fire	finger
fish	four
foot	five

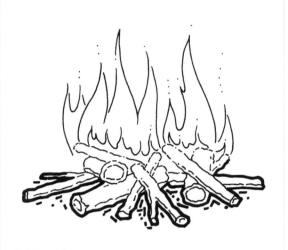

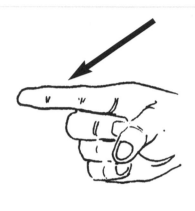

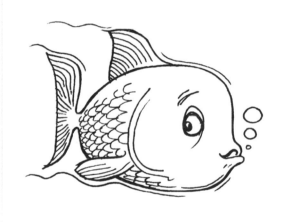

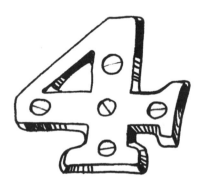

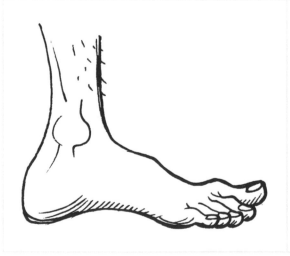

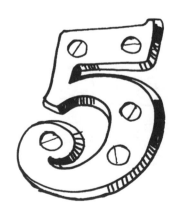

Handout 14 Pictures to elicit articulation of −f

knife	scarf
half	roof
leaf	loaf

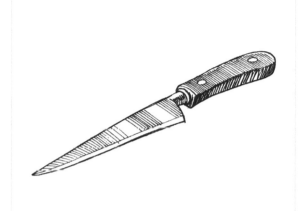 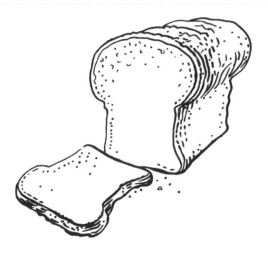

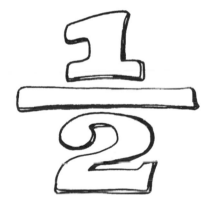 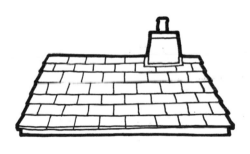

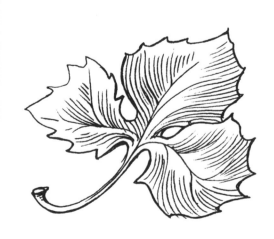 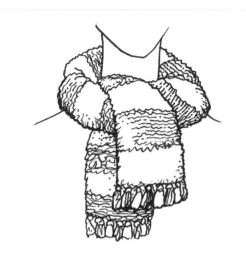

Routledge
Taylor & Francis Group

Handout 15 Pictures to elicit articulation of v–

video	vest
valley	volcano
vase	violin

Handout 16 Pictures to elicit articulation of –v

wave	five
glove	twelve
shave	drive

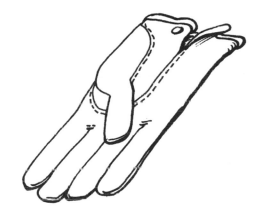 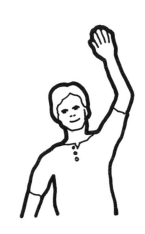 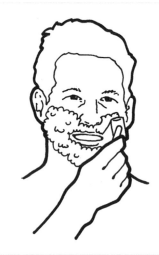

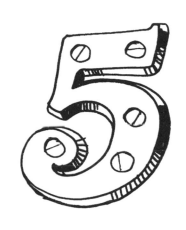 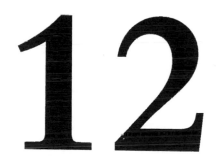 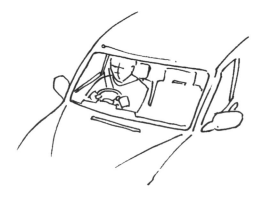

Handout 17 Pictures to elicit articulation of s–

sun	soap
sea	sock
sit	seven

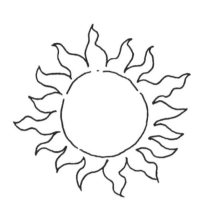

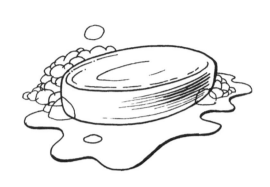

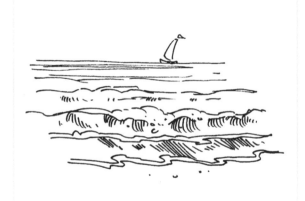

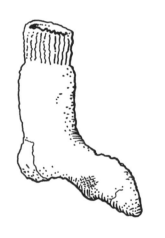

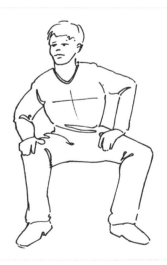

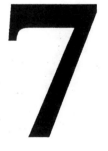

Handout 18 Pictures to elicit articulation of –s

mouse	bus
house	horse
dice	glass

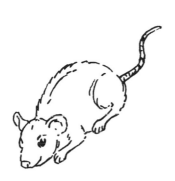

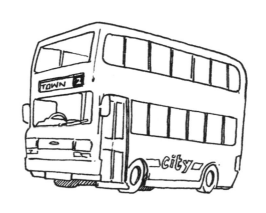

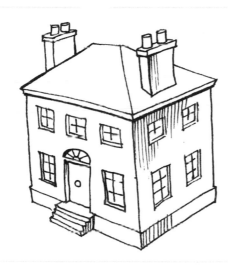

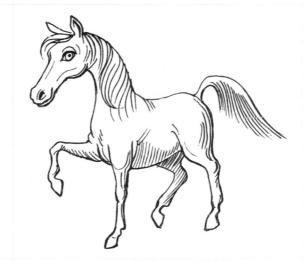

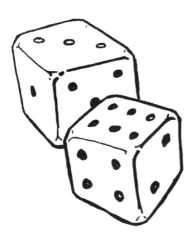

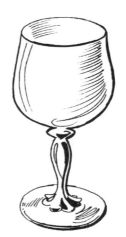

Routledge
Taylor & Francis Group

Handout 19 Pictures to elicit articulation of z–

zero	zoo
zip	zig-zag
z	zebra

Handout 20 Pictures to elicit articulation of –z

buzz	hose
cheese	shoes
nose	cars

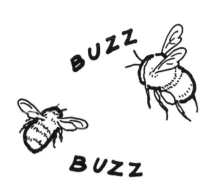

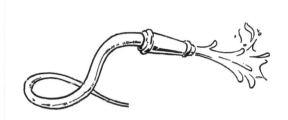

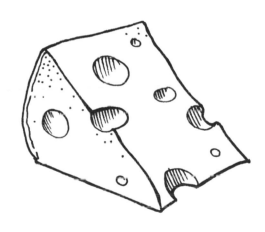

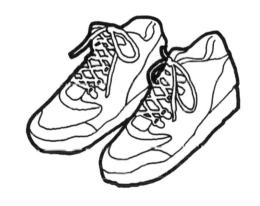

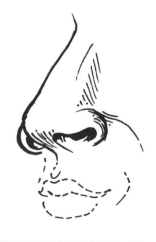

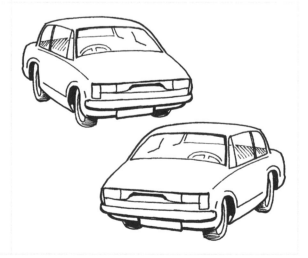

Routledge
Taylor & Francis Group

Handout 21 Pictures to elicit articulation of ʃ–

shoe	sheep
ship	shark
shop	shadow

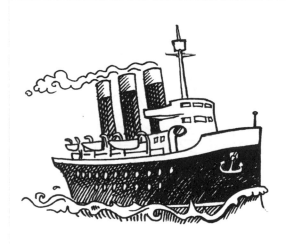

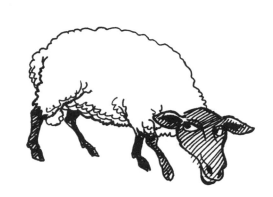

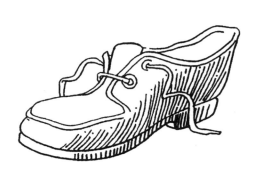

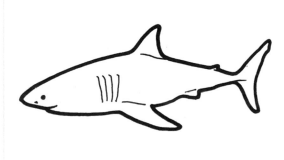

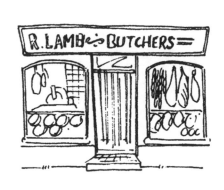

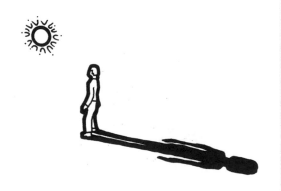

Handout 22 Pictures to elicit articulation of –ʃ

fish	starfish
dish	crash
wash	brush

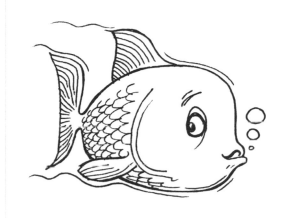

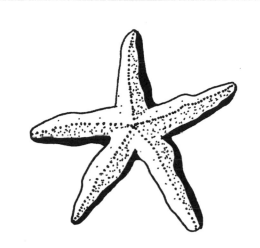

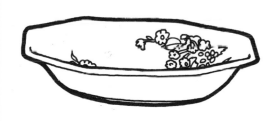

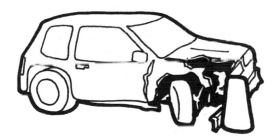

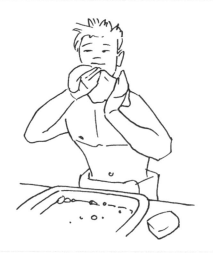

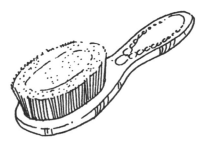

Routledge
Taylor & Francis Group

Handout 23 Pictures to elicit articulation of -ʒ- and -ʒ

measure	rouge
treasure	garage
television	camouflage

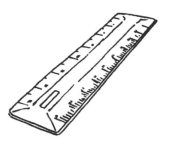

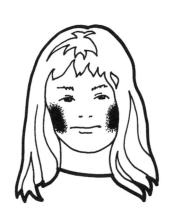

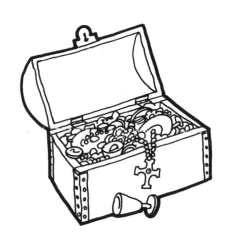

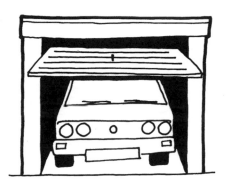

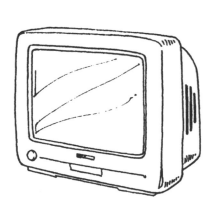

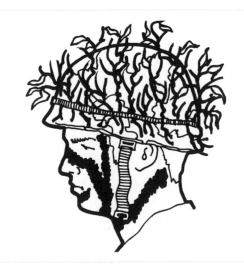

Handout 24 Pictures to elicit articulation of tʃ–

chair	chain
cheese	cherry
chimney	chin

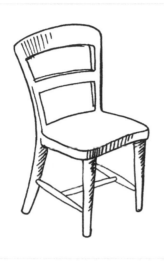
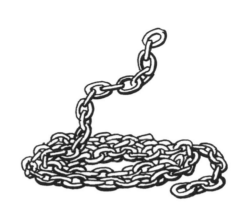

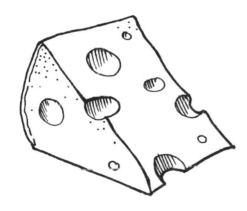
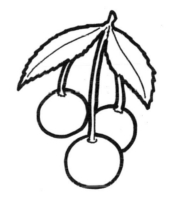

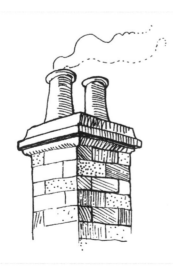
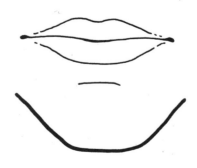

Routledge
Taylor & Francis Group

Handout 25 Pictures to elicit articulation of –tʃ

watch	switch
match	torch
latch	beach

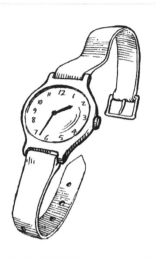

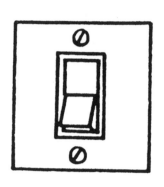

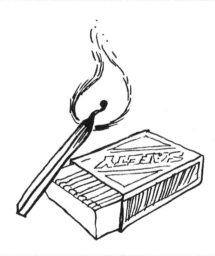

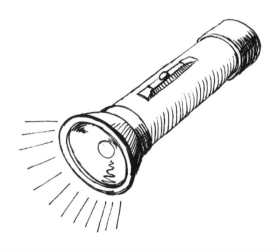

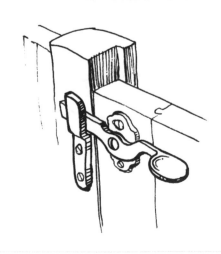

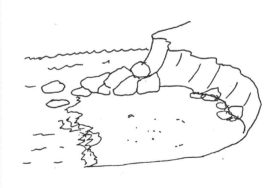

Routledge
Taylor & Francis Group

Handout 26 Pictures to elicit articulation of dʒ-

jam	jersey
jeep	jug
jeans	Jack

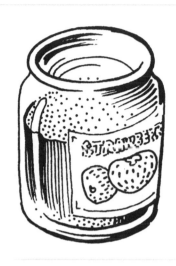
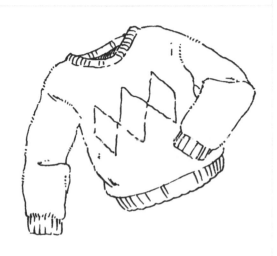

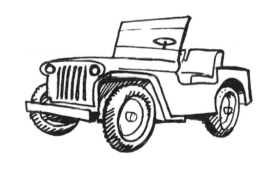
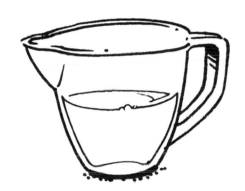

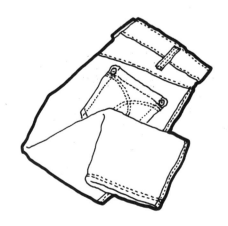
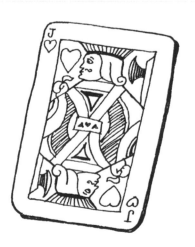

Routledge
Taylor & Francis Group

Handout 27 Pictures to elicit articulation of –dʒ

orange	hedge
bridge	badge
cage	sponge

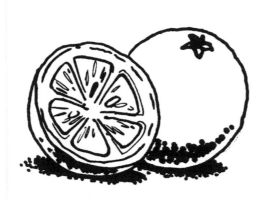

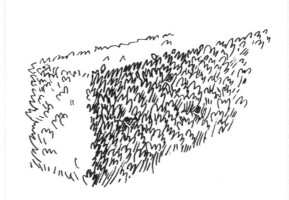

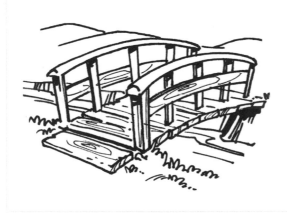

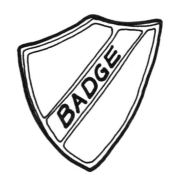

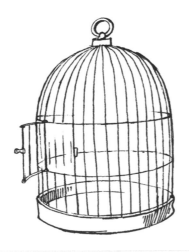

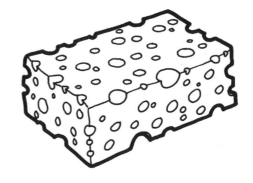

Handout 28 Pictures to elicit articulation of sk–

skip	sky
school	ski
scarf	skirt

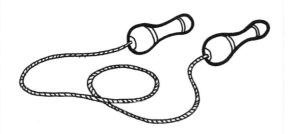

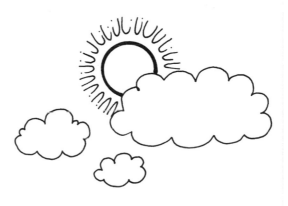

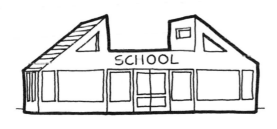

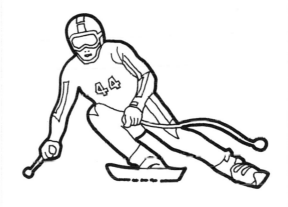

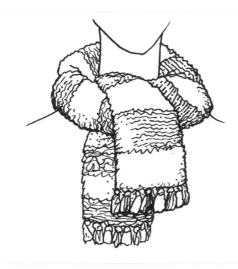

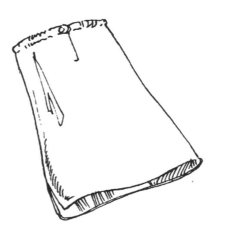

Routledge
Taylor & Francis Group

Handout 29 Pictures to elicit articulation of sp–

spoon	spade
spider	spear
spot	spiral

Handout 30 Pictures to elicit articulation of st–

star	stamp
stop	stair
stool	stick

Handout 31 Pictures to elicit articulation of sm–

smoke	Smarties
smile	smell
small	smart

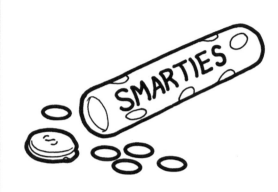

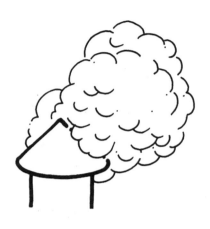

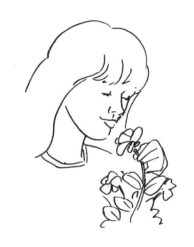

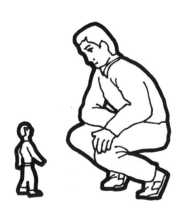

Handout 32 Pictures to elicit articulation of sn–

snail	snore
snake	snowman
snow	snorkel

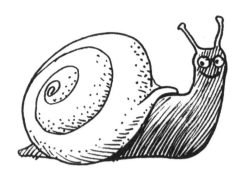

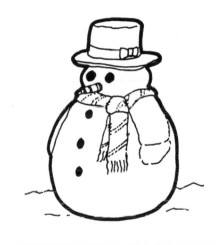

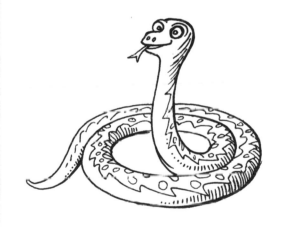

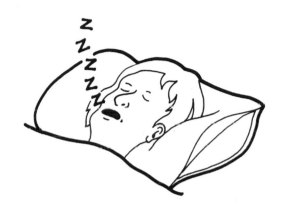

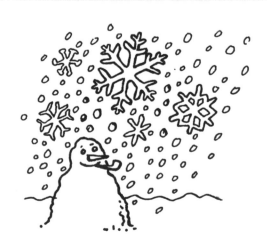

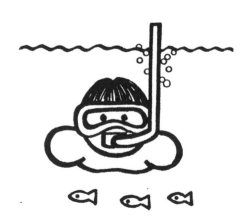

Routledge
Taylor & Francis Group

Handout 33 Pictures to elicit articulation of sl–

slide	sleeve
slipper	sleigh
sleep	slip

Handout 34 Pictures to elicit articulation of sw–

swan	swing
swim	swarm
sweet	swamp

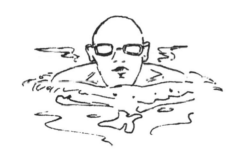
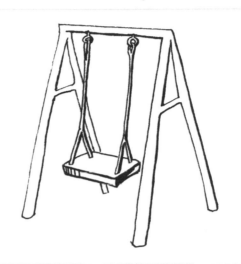
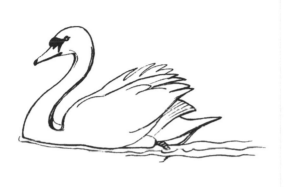
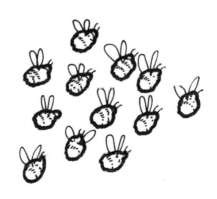
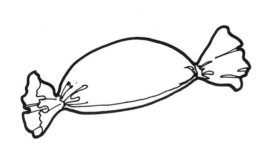
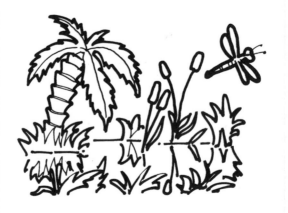

Routledge
Taylor & Francis Group

Handout 35 Single words for practising target sounds

For adults

For adults, reading word lists provide appropriate practice. Some useful single-word lists are reproduced below for target sounds /p, b, t, d, k, g, f, v, s, z, ʃ, ʒ, tʃ, dʒ/ and /s/ clusters.

<table>
<tr><td>/p/</td><td>p–</td><td>–p</td></tr>
<tr><td></td><td>pie</td><td>ape</td></tr>
<tr><td></td><td>pea</td><td>up</td></tr>
<tr><td></td><td>paw</td><td>hip</td></tr>
<tr><td></td><td>pay</td><td>hop</td></tr>
<tr><td></td><td>power</td><td>hope</td></tr>
<tr><td></td><td>pond</td><td>mop</td></tr>
<tr><td></td><td>pipe</td><td>map</td></tr>
<tr><td></td><td>paint</td><td>whip</td></tr>
<tr><td></td><td>paper</td><td>pop</td></tr>
<tr><td></td><td>pain</td><td>pip</td></tr>
<tr><td></td><td>pear</td><td>top</td></tr>
<tr><td></td><td>punch</td><td>tap</td></tr>
<tr><td></td><td>pill</td><td>soup</td></tr>
<tr><td></td><td>pick</td><td>rope</td></tr>
<tr><td></td><td>peach</td><td>heap</td></tr>
</table>

<table>
<tr><td>/b/</td><td>b–</td><td>–b</td></tr>
<tr><td></td><td>buy</td><td>cub</td></tr>
<tr><td></td><td>ball</td><td>bib</td></tr>
<tr><td></td><td>bee</td><td>crab</td></tr>
<tr><td></td><td>bat</td><td>nib</td></tr>
<tr><td></td><td>bit</td><td>knob</td></tr>
<tr><td></td><td>bean</td><td>cob</td></tr>
<tr><td></td><td>bed</td><td>crib</td></tr>
<tr><td></td><td>bike</td><td>hub</td></tr>
<tr><td></td><td>book</td><td>ebb</td></tr>
<tr><td></td><td>bus</td><td>rob</td></tr>
<tr><td></td><td>boat</td><td>fob</td></tr>
<tr><td></td><td>bin</td><td>dab</td></tr>
<tr><td></td><td>ban</td><td>sob</td></tr>
<tr><td></td><td>but</td><td>jab</td></tr>
</table>

<table>
<tr><td>/t/</td><td>t–</td><td>–t</td></tr>
<tr><td></td><td>tea</td><td>eat</td></tr>
<tr><td></td><td>toe</td><td>hat</td></tr>
<tr><td></td><td>tap</td><td>hot</td></tr>
<tr><td></td><td>top</td><td>pot</td></tr>
<tr><td></td><td>type</td><td>pat</td></tr>
<tr><td></td><td>tie</td><td>mat</td></tr>
<tr><td></td><td>tower</td><td>mitt</td></tr>
<tr><td></td><td>tail</td><td>meat</td></tr>
<tr><td></td><td>ten</td><td>neat</td></tr>
<tr><td></td><td>tin</td><td>hit</td></tr>
<tr><td></td><td>tip</td><td>heat</td></tr>
<tr><td></td><td>tear</td><td>pit</td></tr>
<tr><td></td><td>tiny</td><td>sit</td></tr>
<tr><td></td><td>tan</td><td>light</td></tr>
<tr><td></td><td>team</td><td>weight</td></tr>
</table>

<table>
<tr><td>/d/</td><td>d–</td><td>–d</td></tr>
<tr><td></td><td>deer</td><td>red</td></tr>
<tr><td></td><td>Diwali</td><td>road</td></tr>
<tr><td></td><td>dish</td><td>toad</td></tr>
<tr><td></td><td>desk</td><td>food</td></tr>
<tr><td></td><td>door</td><td>wood</td></tr>
<tr><td></td><td>duck</td><td>mud</td></tr>
<tr><td></td><td>dot</td><td>blood</td></tr>
<tr><td></td><td>dirty</td><td>bud</td></tr>
<tr><td></td><td>dog</td><td>rod</td></tr>
<tr><td></td><td>daisy</td><td>lid</td></tr>
<tr><td></td><td>down</td><td>slide</td></tr>
<tr><td></td><td>deep</td><td>wide</td></tr>
<tr><td></td><td>dance</td><td>bed</td></tr>
<tr><td></td><td>dolphin</td><td>bead</td></tr>
<tr><td></td><td>dentist</td><td>sad</td></tr>
</table>

Routledge
Taylor & Francis Group

70

Handout 35 Single words for practising target sounds
continued

/k/	k–	–k
	car	lock
	cup	lick
	cake	rock
	core	back
	carry	look
	can	lake
	cat	ache
	coffee	sick
	cooker	coke
	carpet	duck
	cap	chick
	corn	sock
	cow	rake
	key	kick
	colour	truck

/f/	f–	–f
	fire	knife
	fish	half
	foot	calf
	fee	leaf
	fat	puff
	face	scarf
	fan	laugh
	fight	cough
	fall	rough
	fin	whiff
	four	roof
	five	hoof
	food	safe
	fox	giraffe
	feather	loaf

/g/	g–	–g
	girl	egg
	garage	log
	guy	leg
	goal	wig
	gum	wag
	gear	pig
	gold	big
	gun	bag
	game	flag
	goose	peg
	gate	dig
	guitar	jog
	garden	bug
	goat	rug
	golf	hug

/v/	v–	–v
	video	give
	valley	wave
	vat	love
	vase	glove
	vowel	mauve
	Vicky	live
	voice	move
	veil	shave
	vest	cave
	vegetable	sleeve
	village	hive
	vein	dive
	volcano	twelve
	valentine	five
	violin	dove

Routledge
Taylor & Francis Group

71

/s/	s–	–s
	sun	horse
	sand	house
	sea	grass
	soup	mouse
	sit	dice
	sieve	cross
	six	ice
	sofa	face
	seagull	lace
	sock	moss
	sum	mice
	salt	miss
	seven	hiss
	saw	nice
	sink	glass

/z/	z–	–z
	zebra	buzz
	zoo	cheese
	xylophone	nose
	zig-zag	rose
	zero	eggs
	zinc	bees
	zip	hose
	zany	flies
	zap	jars
	zoom	shoes
	Z	sneeze
	zeal	fizz
	zest	whizz
	zodiac	Liz
	zone	fuzz

/ʃ/	ʃ–	–ʃ
	shoe	fish
	shower	dish
	shampoo	wash
	sharp	rash
	ship	wish
	sheep	mesh
	sugar	crash
	shoot	crush
	sheet	brush
	shop	blush
	shark	rush
	shy	push
	shave	bush
	shovel	splosh
	shepherd	splash

/ʒ/	–ʒ–	–ʒ
	measure	ménage
	treasure	beige
	pleasure	rouge
	television	garage (may be /dʒ/)
	usual	barrage
	Asian (may be /sh/)	prestige
	division	mirage
	collision	camouflage
	leisure	sabotage

Routledge
Taylor & Francis Group

Handout 35 Single words for practising target sounds
continued

/tʃ / tʃ–	–tʃ
chair	watch
chapati	match
chip	church
cheque	witch
chin	arch
child	catch
children	bench
chicken	torch
chop	hutch
chest	beach
cherry	branch
chain	pitch
cheese	leach
chocolate	peach
chimney	ditch

/dʒ/ dʒ–	–dʒ
jam	garage (may be /ʒ/)
jeep	porridge
jeans	fridge
jockey	orange
jersey	sponge
jump	luggage
jug	page
juggler	bridge
jacket	cage
giant	badge
jelly	hedge
Jack	George
joke	cabbage
jewel	sausage
giraffe	wedge

Routledge Taylor & Francis Group P This page may be photocopied for instructional use only. *Practical Intervention for Cleft Palate Speech* © Jane Russell & Liz Albery 2005

/s/ clusters	sk–	sp–	st–
	skate	spoon	star
	ski	spider	stick
	school	spot	stop
	skip	spade	stair
	scarf	spoil	stoop
	skirt	space	station
	scatter	speed	steer
	Scotland	spike	stump
	scary	spear	stamp
	scamp	spiral	stool
	sky	spill	stuck

sm–	sn–	sl–	sw–
smoke	snail	slide	swan
smile	snout	slip	swim
small	sniff	slippery	sweet
smooth	sneeze	slipper	swarm
Smarties	snooze	sleep	swot
smirk	snake	sleeve	swamp
smatter	snore	slam	swallow
smart	sneak	slow	swell
smother	snap	slop	swollen
smell	snow	sleigh	swipe
smitten	snatch	sleet	swine

Handout 36 Short sentences for practising target sounds

Any single word from the word lists can be incorporated into short sentences.

/p–/	/–p/
1 Put the paper away.	1 Turn on the tap.
2 Peter is a nice boy.	2 The soap was slippery.
3 Mum makes lots of pies.	3 I bought sweets at the shop.
4 Pigs live in a sty.	4 He wore a blue cap.
5 Poi's dress is pink.	5 She looked at the map.

/b–/	/–b/
1 The baby is asleep.	1 A little fox cub.
2 Kick the ball.	2 He wore a bib.
3 Wheel him in the buggy.	3 The spider made a web.
4 He's saying bye-bye.	4 The car hit the kerb.
5 Beth is five.	5 His name is Bob.

/t–/	/–t/
1 I hurt my toe.	1 The rain made everything wet.
2 Tea is nearly ready.	2 A black cat is lucky.
3 Take a taxi.	3 She wore a huge hat.
4 Don't tip it over.	4 The gate opened.
5 Tell me the time.	5 Please sit still.

/d–/	/–d/
1 Do you like sweets?	1 Dig with a spade.
2 The donkey was very old.	2 Peter went to bed.
3 Ajit likes to dance.	3 He grew a black beard.
4 She's afraid of the dark.	4 The car slid on the ice.
5 Some people play darts.	5 There was a bend in the road.

/k–/	/–k/
1 Kangaroos can travel fast.	1 The duck was green and brown.
2 You need a windy day to fly a kite.	2 She lost a sock.
3 Tom had a Mickey mouse cake.	3 The air was filled with smoke.
4 She gave the baby a kiss.	4 He felt very sick.
5 He took a photo with his camera.	5 They played in the park.

This page may be photocopied for instructional use only. *Practical Intervention for Cleft Palate Speech* © Jane Russell & Liz Albery 2005

Page 1 of 3

/g-/	/-g/
1 The car is in the garage.	1 The hen laid an egg.
2 He scored a goal.	2 The judge wore a wig.
3 A pretty garden.	3 He was a big baby.
4 They won the game.	4 Give Mummy a hug.
5 She played the guitar.	5 Dig the garden.

/f-/	/-f/
1 Cod is a type of fish.	1 Cut with a knife.
2 She had very big feet.	2 A baby cow is a calf.
3 Please fetch your shoes.	3 He climbed onto the roof.
4 Her father gave her four coins.	4 A giraffe has a very long neck.
5 A fan kept them cool.	5 The leaf was golden brown.

/v-/	/-v/
1 He watched a cartoon DVD.	1 Safian gave her a diamond ring.
2 They skied into the valley.	2 That was a close shave!
3 Jane played the violin well.	3 They had five children.
4 Postman Pat drives a van.	4 He left a glove behind.
5 She doesn't like wearing a vest.	5 Could you give me more time?

/s-/	/-s/
1 The sun shone all day.	1 They played tennis.
2 Pam felt a bit sad.	2 The bus was late.
3 She wished he would sit still.	3 The grass had grown very long.
4 Use some soap to wash your hands.	4 He was crazy about tomato sauce.
5 John was nearly six years old.	5 The police chased the joy rider.

/z-/	/-z/
1 A zebra has black and white stripes.	1 Bees make honey.
2 There were lions at the zoo.	2 He collected jam jars.
3 Sue broke her zip.	3 She loved red shoes.
4 He played the xylophone.	4 Grandpa watered the garden with a hose.
5 The lightning made a zig-zag in the sky.	5 A tickle in his nose made him sneeze.

Handout 36 Short sentences for practising target sounds
continued

/ʃ-/

1 Show me the way please.
2 Do you like a bath or a shower?
3 Some men hate shaving.
4 Sharks can be scary.
5 Too much sugar is bad for you.

/-ʃ/

1 Have you ever caught a fish?
2 He threw a coin and made a wish.
3 Mum told the dirty children to have a wash.
4 David broke the dish.
5 A fire burns down to ash.

/-ʒ-/

1 He found the treasure at last.
2 Dad took the children to a pleasure park.
3 He used a tape to measure.

/-ʒ/

1 Lock up the garage.
2 She wore a beige dress.
3 A camouflage jacket.

/tʃ-/

1 Sit on the chair.
2 We saw chimps at the zoo.
3 Most people like fish and chips.
4 He had a hairy chest.
5 Tom likes cherry pie.

/-tʃ/

1 Jane looked at her watch.
2 The little boy tried to catch the ball.
3 It was a good tennis match.
4 The rabbit lived in a big wooden hutch.
5 Soldiers often march.

/dʒ-/

1 Mum likes strawberry jam.
2 He was always playing jokes.
3 Jeans are very useful.
4 He liked to be called George.
5 She drives a black jeep.

/-dʒ/

1 The hedge needs trimming.
2 She sat on the edge of her seat.
3 He ate a big wedge of cheese.
4 We need a new fridge.
5 The bridge went over the river.

Practical Intervention for Cleft Palate Speech © Jane Russell & Liz Albery 2005

Routledge
Taylor & Francis Group

Generalisation

It is difficult to predict exactly when a child or adult will generalise to his everyday speech the work that he has done in therapy. This is because generalisation is subject to many variables, such as motivation, self-monitoring skills and the amount of support given by parents, relatives, friends and teachers.

Many teachers know very little about cleft lip and palate, and the therapist may find it helpful to give them an 'Advice for teachers' handout (see Appendix 3), which covers basic facts about cleft lip and palate, hearing, hospitalisation and teasing/bullying; this may be photocopied. Some children and adults generalise work learnt very quickly. Others take months, or even years.

In pre-school children

Very young children often generalise quite quickly, presumably because of fewer years of habit. Ideas for generalisation may include describing pictures, trying to remember one sound (such as /s/) correctly, and then progressing to more than one sound to remember.

Parents may be asked to help the process of generalisation by gently encouraging correct use of whichever consonant sounds the therapist feels the child is ready to generalise. If it is felt that it would be too much to correct a child all day long, it is worthwhile in the initial stages to choose a certain period of the day, such as teatime or bathtime, when a child is expected to remember his 'good' speech. Puppets and dolls can be used to listen to a child, to ask them whether they said the word correctly, or to give them the correct model. There is a fine line between not bothering to correct a child at all and nagging them so much that they communicate less freely.

For younger children in particular, lots of positive feedback is essential and the generous use of stars, stickers and badges goes down well! Any nursery staff should be made aware of sounds that the therapist feels a child should be ready to generalise. Although they probably will not have time to work individually with a child, they have a useful role in monitoring generalisation, may be able to encourage correct use of sounds when speaking one-to-one and may even instigate project work to emphasise a certain sound. For example, for /s/ a project on the seaside can be helpful and may include words such as *sun, sand, seagull, spade, sunglasses, sandwich* and so on.

In the speech and language therapy clinic

Picture description is helpful. The therapist can agree with the child which sound(s) to concentrate on and can use a stopwatch to monitor the length of time the child can speak without making a mistake. A chart can then be filled in, with the times taken. This seems to focus children's minds on the task.

At home

Reading out loud is good practice for sound generalisation and for five- to eight-year-old children a school reading book is helpful. This can easily form part of a home therapy programme. Recording conversation topics and playing them back so that the child can point out his own 'mistakes' can be a valuable aid to self-monitoring. Topics could include 'My School', 'My Friends', 'Different Sports', 'My Favourite TV Programme (or Advertisement)', 'Computer Games' and 'My Favourite Holiday would be ...'. An incentive chart using stars or stickers may be useful, as may a 'Progress Chart', which can be blocked in by the child. For ideas of other reward systems see Chapter 6. See Table 3 for an example programme of therapy for a child aged five years.

Adults may have to combat many years of incorrect consonant production and their degree of motivation and effort is crucial during this stage (see Chapter 7). It is helpful for an adult to read a newspaper or book out loud, having agreed with the therapist which consonants he is going to pronounce correctly. When reading is 100 per cent or almost 100 per cent correct, the therapist can move on to recording short conversations with the client and playing them back so that together they may identify any errors.

Case example

Session plan for Asif

Table 3 on page 80 shows a typical session plan for a child aged five years. Assessment showed production of /t/ as /?/ and /s/ as /x/ in all positions.

After session 3, Asif, who had very supportive parents, went away for one month to practise everything from this session. Review after one month became review at three months until the therapist was sure that generalisation had taken place.

TABLE 3 Session plan for Asif, aged five years

Plan	Activity	Method & Materials
Session 1 (45 minutes) **Aim** To target consonant /t/.	Check discrimination and recognition of /t/ versus /ʔ/ then attempt labiodental /t/. Obtained labiodental /t/ and practised until stable. Asked child to move the labiodental /t/ back behind teeth. This was successful and VC combinations /iːt/, /aːt/ were obtained. Encouraged to practise at home.	Therapist imitates correct/ incorrect production of /t/ in words and scores child's discrimination and recognition. /t/ needs to be 100% correct in isolation. Used a mirror for visual feedback. Used Black Sheep pictures for VC combinations (/t/ initial and final).
Session 2 (One hour) **Aims** To begin with /t/ final in words, then /t/ initial in words; if possible to introduce /s/ in isolation.	Introduced word-final /t/. This was easy, then tried word-initial /t/. An intrusive glottal appeared, /tʔiː/. Tried /t–hiː/ gently then phased /h/ out. Even though /t/ initial not yet firmly established we used /t/ in isolation as a facilitator for /s/, that is /tsssssssss/ explaining that we wanted to produce a very long /t/. This was then used word-finally as in *bets, mats*. Unlike /t/ initial the child was able to then integrate /s/ successfully in word-initial position. Asked to practise /t/ and /s/ at single word level at home.	Used Black Sheep pictures (/t/ initial and final). Played the Clapa Thameside games to practise /t/ and /s/. Used sheets as above and then to move out of 'drill' mode played Clapa Thameside games for /t/ and /s/. Black Sheep pictures were copied for home use.
Session 3 (45 minutes) **Aims** To check production of /t/ and /s/ in single words; if successful move on to words in short sentences.	Checked on production of /t/ and /s/ in single words, which was fine. Made up a list of 'Keywords'. Put /t/ and /s/ into short sentences and encouraged self-monitoring.	Used the computer for keywords. Used record and playback so the child could start to pick out his own errors.

Approaches used with Articulation Therapy and Remediation of Specific Cleft-type Characteristics

5

Approaches used with articulation therapy

Therapy for children with cleft palate is essentially an eclectic approach, and aspects of the following techniques can be useful when used alongside articulation therapy.

Phonological therapy

As Russell and Harding (2001) describe, once a new articulatory target is being produced accurately and consistently, phonological techniques can help to establish it in different word positions and facilitate generalisation (Grunwell & Dive, 1988; Grundy & Harding, 1995; Russell & Sell, 1998).

Consonant recognition and discrimination activities have been described in Chapter 3. Following on from these discrimination activities, children learn to sort and produce words according to phonemic contrasts; for example, words beginning with /t/ versus /k/, or words ending in /tʃ/, /ʃ/, /f/ or /s/. Minimal pairs may be used to help children convey different meaning, as in homophony confrontation (Grunwell & Dive, 1988). Pairs games, sentences, picture description, rhymes and conversation also provide opportunities for target consonants to be used in meaningful contexts.

Pairs games

These will be very familiar to therapists. A set of pictures containing two of each picture is placed face down on the table. One player turns over two pictures and names them (with the target accurately produced, of course!). If the pictures are identical, the player keeps the pair and has another go. If they are different, the pictures are replaced face down and it is the next player's turn. The game can be used to demand lots of repetitions of target consonants within words and can be made harder by requiring the player to use the word accurately in a sentence before being allowed to 'win' the pair. Examples of these games can be seen on the GOS-CLAPA Therapy Video (see Appendix 4).

Minimal pairs

Words that differ by one consonant are selected. For example, for a child who is backing to velar but is now able to produce /t/ accurately, words such as *tea – key*, *ten – Ken*, *tall – call* and so on would be selected. If the therapist wished to work on the contrast at the ends of words, then words such as *bat – back*, *rat – rack*, *bite – bike* would be chosen. The words can either be represented as pictures or, for older children who can read, they can be written. Games are constructed in which the child has to use the correct word to convey meaning at a simple single word level at first and then in sentences and stories in order to make the task more difficult.

Metaphon

In some instances, articulation and phonological therapy approaches may be supported by the use of *Metaphon* (Howell & Dean, 1994). *Metaphon* aims to increase children's knowledge of language and communication by providing a specific learning environment. The increase in knowledge is then used to 'enhance communicative ability' (Howell & Dean, 1994).

Howell and Dean (1994) describe the adaptation of *Metaphon* by Harland, so that it may be used with cleft palate children alongside articulation therapy. It can help to label the contrasts that are being targeted, for example 'front' versus 'back' consonants (Russell & Sell, 1998). The contrasts between oral, nasal and glottal productions may be illustrated using the concepts of Mr Mouth, Mr Nose and Mr Throat.

Cued articulation

Cued Articulation (Passy, 1990) is a system of simple hand signs which are used to help children remember consonants. They can be used by the therapist to provide visual cues and by the child to help him to remember the required articulatory movements. An example is the placing of the index finger vertically with the end of the finger close to one side of the lips and moving it forward as the sound /t/ is made. This helps the child remember that the front of the tongue should be used and that the required consonant is a plosive.

Use of instrumentation in therapy

Electropalatography

Although electropalatography (EPG) has been around for some time, it is only since the late 1990s that it has become accepted generally in cleft palate centres as a therapeutic tool. The aim of EPG is to provide visual feedback of tongue positioning for sounds. An individual plate is made for the palate and contact points are inserted strategically throughout the plate. The plate is then placed in the mouth and connected to a PC, which gives a visual display of where the tongue is contacting the palate. Fiona Gibbon at the University of Edinburgh is currently researching the efficacy of EPG; meanwhile, therapists are reporting success and rapid progress when it is used with some clients. For a supplier see Appendix 4.

Speech Viewer III

Speech Viewer III is useful for some speech sound production tasks such as phoneme accuracy: it allows clients to practise making sounds in isolation. If a target is reached an animation is shown. It is easy to use. For a supplier see Appendix 4.

For a list of selected software applications to assist therapy please see Appendix 4.

Remediation of specific cleft-type characteristics

Backing

Backing is a systemic phonological simplification that is the opposite of the normal fronting process (Grunwell, 1985). It usually involves, the realisation of target alveolar consonants as velars, for example /t/ → /k/, /d/ → /g/, but, as indicated on the *GOS.SP.ASS.98* form (Sell *et al*, 1999), 'Backing to uvular' is also a possible posterior oral cleft-type characteristic. Backing may occur in the presence of a fistula, when it is thought to be related to the fact that pressure can be built up more easily behind the fistula. However, a preference for back articulation has also been noted in the developing speech of children with cleft palate who do not have fistulae (Russell & Grunwell, 1993, Russell & Harding, 2001). If backing is detected during assessment, the therapist needs to be alert to the possibility of it affecting any alveolar consonants, including nasals and laterals. These may require specific remediation.

Therapy

Therapy to remediate a backing pattern involves both articulatory and phonological approaches. Articulatory approaches will establish accurate production of the target alveolar consonant; phonological approaches will help the child understand how the target differs from his habitual production and affects the meaning of what he is trying to say.

Care needs to be taken when teaching a child to produce alveolar plosives in particular because of the danger of developing double articulation. For this reason, as with other targets, the child should be able to produce the sound accurately and easily, both in isolation and in consonant sequences, before attempting to use it in meaningful words. For some children, phonetic explanations with the aid of diagrams may be helpful, as well as visual and tactile feedback.

Techniques for eliciting /t/ and /d/ are described on page 31. In cases where it is proving difficult not to inhibit the velar it might help to start from the interdental /th/, instructing the child to put his tongue out as far as he can. This can then be turned into an exaggerated dental /t/ or /d/. Parents may need to be reassured about this strange production! Clinical experience has shown that once a fronted target is achieved and drilled, a more natural articulation develops over time.

At the same time as learning production strategies, the child should be taught to identify 'front' versus 'back' consonants. Young children enjoy listening to sounds made by the therapist or parent and placing counters on the front or back of a crocodile's mouth. At first the stimulus will be a sound produced in isolation but as the child's ability to identify the sound improves the task can be made harder by asking the child to listen for the sound in a syllable or in a particular word position.

When the child is able to produce an acceptable alveolar production and can contrast it with his velar production in isolation and in words, therapy becomes more phonologically based. Minimal pairs can be used in games to encourage the child to maintain the contrast in his speech in order to convey different meanings.

Eliminating glottal stops

This is another area of therapy where care needs to be taken to establish consistent production of the target consonant before making any attempt to include it in words. Otherwise there is a danger of the child producing the target consonant with simultaneous glottal articulation or glottal reinforcement.

Therapy

In order to inhibit the glottal stop the vocal folds need to be kept apart, which can be achieved by whispering, over aspiration or the use of a sustained /h/. Golding-Kushner (2001) recommends starting therapy with /h/ 'to establish production of an oral airflow with an open glottis'. To eliminate glottal stops the sustained /h/ is overlaid with labial or lingual gestures. An alternative method also advocated by Golding-Kushner is to whisper plosive sounds with over aspiration, then introduce voicing at the end of the syllable with a gradual shift of the voice onset time.

Similarly, Harding and Grunwell (1998) suggest that 'Use of soft attack similar to gentle whisper for all target models ensures minimal articulatory effort'. Another useful technique proposed by these authors is to stretch the duration of segment transitions in VC and CV models. This works well when hand stroking is used, see page 27.

Lateralisation

A degree of lateralisation is a common cleft-type characteristic. Missing lateral incisor(s) may predispose a client to the feature of lateralisation, as, possibly, may a narrowed maxillary arch.

Therapy

For the older child or adult, the therapist can explain that the sides of the tongue should contact the upper side teeth and the tongue tip should be raised (or, for some people, lowered) with a groove in the middle for the airstream to travel. With most children, the therapist can use a straw placed centrally on the tongue and the child can try to blow through this for /s/, making some bubbles in a glass of water (if the airstream is not central, no bubbles will appear). Another method is to obtain /s/ from a long /t/, backwards from a /θ/ or forwards from a /ʃ/ (see Table 2, page 31). It seems that where lateralisation is resistant to change, and traditional methods of remediation have been tried, EPG may be a successful option (see page 83).

Working in the presence of suspected or confirmed velopharyngeal dysfunction

As described with regard to influencing factors, it can be beneficial and often important to continue to work towards accurate articulation and manner of production even when velopharyngeal dysfunction is suspected or confirmed. The only time when this is not necessary is where normal articulation patterns have developed and, although there is hypernasality and/or audible nasal emission, the client has intelligible speech.

Therapy

As Golding-Kushner (2001) and Sell and Grunwell (2001) explain, specific exercises intended to improve palate function and, therefore, achieve velopharyngeal closure are not appropriate and do not work. Only when the patient has been shown to be capable of achieving velopharyngeal closure during a speech task, usually from nasopharyngoscopy or multiview videofluoroscopy, may some therapy be indicated. Ideally this would be visual biofeedback using nasopharyngoscopy, but therapy focusing on awareness and production of oral versus nasal consonants may be helpful.

Young children respond well to the concept of sounds produced by 'Mr Mouth' or 'Mr Nose' (see Appendix 1), whereas older children and adults can be taught more specifically about how the target consonants are produced. In both instances, visual prompts using pictures and phonetic diagrams are used.

Active nasal fricatives

The distinction between active and passive nasal fricatives is an important one for management. The difference between active and passive has been well-described by Harding and Grunwell (1998). Essentially, an active nasal fricative assumes the physical potential for correct production of the consonant(s) affected, with speech therapy being the management procedure of choice. A passive nasal fricative is caused by underlying velopharyngeal insufficiency, which is most likely to be remediated by surgery.

In the past, some children with active nasal fricatives have had surgery inappropriately and post-surgery the habit of articulating nasally sounds such as /s/ and /z/ remains. This is not to say that a child with active nasal fricatives should *never* undergo surgery for VPI, because VPI may be present throughout speech in addition to the presence of active nasal fricatives.

We can only speculate as to why some children acquire the habit of active nasal fricatives. One possible theory is that as the majority of these children have a history of middle ear effusions they mis-hear fricatives in particular at a crucial early stage and learn to articulate these sounds nasally. It is also true that many of these children have had a cleft palate or submucous cleft and possibly an underlying palate weakness plus hearing difficulties: these conditions predispose children to acquire this particular pattern of speech.

Any or all fricatives and affricates may be misarticulated as active nasal fricatives. Typically the /s/ and /z/ consonants are most frequently affected, and commonly /f, v, ʃ, ʒ, tʃ, dʒ/. It is interesting to note that in the authors' experience the affricates, which are acquired later in developmental terms, are sometimes correctly articulated when /s/, acquired earlier, is not. Generally the pattern of nasal fricatives is consistent and consonants both in initial and final positions in words are affected. Occasionally there is an obvious variability in production – perhaps a final /s/ is realised as /t/, or it may be correctly realised. This tells us that the child's sound system is already in the process of change, and should make some stages of therapy easier.

Assessment

Assessment should follow the same process as for any other cleft-related speech difficulty. Use *CAPS-A* (John *et al*, in press) or *GOS.SP.ASS* (Sell *et al*, 1994, 1999). If a child is presenting for the first time at the age of between three and five years, with no past history of a palate problem, it is unlikely that hypernasality suggestive of VPI will be noted. The active nasal fricatives are therefore present as an obvious cleft-type characteristic rather than a sign of general VPI. Quite often developmental immaturities will also be noted as a less severe problem in the speech sound system of these children. For children with a history of cleft palate, active nasal fricatives may exist as just one cleft-type characteristic among others, for example backing (see page 83).

Therapy

Therapy follows the same principles as described in Chapter 4.

1 Eliciting consonants in isolation (aim to achieve 100 per cent correct production in isolation and sequences of consonants)
2 Eliciting CV and VC combinations (in nonsense syllables)
3 Eliciting single words
4 Eliciting short sentences
5 Generalisation.

Some stages are more difficult than others and a number of factors will influence the therapy progress and outcome (see Chapter 1). For this group of children, many of whom have had and continue to have hearing difficulties, it is not ideal to embark on a programme of therapy when hearing levels are down.

Once-weekly therapy can be very prolonged, so best results are obtained from an initial prolonged or intensive session. A two-hour morning session broken into three or four chunks is generally very productive in allowing plenty of time to practise the production of one or two consonants in isolation, nonsense syllables and single words. It may only be necessary to run one session of this length, depending on the child's motivation and other factors, such as the number of consonants affected. Frequently it is the specialist speech and language therapists working in the cleft centres who are able to undertake this length of session, and often a child can then be referred back to the local therapist for any follow-up therapy. Link and local therapists can obtain good results from therapy for active nasal fricatives, but given their demanding caseloads, it is sometimes difficult for them to book only one child per morning for therapy. If there is more than one child in a therapist's caseload with active nasal fricatives, some group intensive therapy (for example, two hours a day for four days) can be effective, particularly as a motivator.

Motivation is very important. This type of therapy requires good concentration levels and a wish to succeed. Sometimes a child who is unconcerned that his speech is different and that people have difficulty understanding him, will see therapy as irrelevant to him. At times therefore, despite pressure from parents and school, it is necessary to wait a while until a child is ready to co-operate in clinic and to practise between therapy sessions. There is a lot of variability in this readiness for therapy, with some children ready at three or four years of age, and some much later.

Difficult stages in therapy

Eliciting consonants in isolation

Probably the elicitation of consonants in isolation causes most difficulty. Use Table 2 in Chapter 4 to target individual consonants. Most frequently /s/ is elicited from a prolonged /t/. Remember to teach the consonant as if it is a new sound to try to avoid the habit factor.

Eliciting single words and VC / CV combinations

Another stage that can be difficult is the integration of the target consonant word initially, as in *s-un*. Some children integrate it easily; others produce the correct target consonant then produce an intrusive nasal fricative before the vowel. This sometimes happens because the therapist is trying to move on to single words too soon. Target consonants need to be 100 per cent correct in isolation and consonant sequences. For a time, which may vary from one to a few sessions, it may be necessary to separate the /s/ from the rest of the word to inhibit the intrusive nasal fricative. Word final is generally much easier, so when introducing a new consonant sound into words start with word final. Use the hand stroking technique to encourage prolonged /s/, and continuous sound into the vowel facilitates VC and CV syllables: /s::i/ and /i::s/. Another way of facilitating this is to add in /h/ to avoid a break and discourage an intrusive nasal, for example /s–hi/, /s–ha/.

Generalisation

Generalisation of the new sound into everyday speech can also be difficult and varies greatly from child to child, some generalising very quickly and others taking many months. Successful generalisation depends on a number of factors, such as motivation, level of practice, phonological maturity and the ability of a child to monitor his own speech. For specific ideas on encouraging generalisation, see Chapter 4.

Case example

Session plan for Jack

Jack, aged five years, presented with a pattern of active nasal fricatives, some developmental errors and a history of middle-ear effusions with episodes of otitis media. His speech was not always intelligible and comments were starting about his speech from his peers at school. Difficulties with his presenting sound system consisted of /s, z, f, v/ being articulated as nasal fricatives. In addition /k, g/ was realised as /t, d/ (fronting) and clusters were reduced. Jack was also unable to imitate /s, z, f, v/ correctly in isolation.

An initial morning of therapy was arranged and the therapy programme shown in Table 4 was devised.

Once new consonant sounds were established easily in clinic in all word positions, Jack needed to practise daily at home. A list of key words for Jack was helpful in starting the process of generalisation into everyday games; in addition this list included frequently used words such as *Please, School*. Further ideas for generalisation can be found in Chapter 4.

TABLE 4 Session plan for Jack, aged five years

Plan	Activity	Materials
Session 1 (2 hours in chunks of 30 minutes) to target /f/ and /s/ in isolation; to obtain /f/ and /s/ in word final position.	Obtained /f/ first as most visual using the *Nuffield Dyspraxia Programme Firework* representation. Obtained /s/ from prolonged /t/. No problem with either in word-final position.	*Nuffield Dyspraxia Programme* sheets; Black Sheep sheets; Speech Viewer III.
Practice sheets (eg, *Nuffield Dyspraxia Programme* and Black Sheep) given to take home for 2 weeks.		
Session 2 (45 minutes) to target /f, s/ in word-initial position; to introduce /v, z/ in isolation and in single words.	Unable to obtain smooth integration of /f, s/ syllable or word-initial. Introduced /h/ between the /f/ and /s/ initial and the following vowel, for example /f–ha/, /s–hi/. /v/ easier than /z/. Again unable to obtain smooth integration word-initially and inserted /h/.	CV nonsense syllables in Black Sheep: /f, s/ initial.

Black Sheep sheets; Speech Viewer III |
| Practice sheets taken home for 2 weeks. | | |
| | | Following Session 2 and short periods of daily practice, Jack successfully integrated /f, s/ word-initially. |

Providing the Client with Practice and Support

The importance of ensuring that support is available to the client has already been discussed with regard to influencing factors and maintaining motivation (see Chapter 1). It is also closely linked to the understanding of therapy objectives and the effectiveness of different models of service delivery.

Consistent 'daily' practice – whose responsibility?

Even when a period of intensive therapy can be provided, regular daily home practice is important. If therapy is only weekly or less frequent, daily practice is essential if changes in speech are to be achieved and maintained. Golding-Kushner (1995) recommends that 'regardless of where therapy is provided, 10 minutes of home practice should be scheduled on non therapy days with homework assignments written into a speech notebook'. She also discusses the responsibilities of the therapist, the parent and the client, and suggests that a formal written contract signed by all parties may be useful.

- Therapist's responsibility – 'to keep the parent informed about the therapy process and impose involvement in therapy on the parent'.
- Parent's responsibility – 'to be aware of current target sounds and contexts and the therapy procedures, so that they can continue the therapy programme at home'.
- Patient's responsibility – 'to participate actively in therapy and home practice tasks.'

Golding-Kushner (1995)

As discussed above, the therapist's responsibilities may be time-consuming, particularly if the child is seen in a school setting with the parent not usually present. However, time invested in explanation to the parent and in ensuring that homework is carried out in the right way means that the therapy programme is likely to be more effective and time-efficient overall. In particular it helps to prevent the frustrations experienced by everyone when progress is not being made.

Who else could help?

In situations where it is difficult to achieve the type of 'contract' advocated by Golding-Kushner (1995), and if the parent or carer is unable to carry out regular home practice for whatever reason, it is important for the therapist to take time to identify other sources of support.

For children attending nursery or school, this may be a particular person within that environment. This could be an identified individual specifically funded by the school or local education authority (LEA) to help children with special needs. In most situations, however, participation relies on the goodwill of the teaching staff and classroom assistants. Once again, it is important for the therapist to take time to provide explanation and demonstration, so that any activities are directly related to the child's needs. Unfortunately, general programmes aimed at children with delayed speech and language development are not appropriate. As described earlier in this book, children with cleft palate-related speech difficulties require specific focused articulation therapy. However, the practice need not be time-consuming or onerous; for example, it may be sufficient that the child produces 20 productions of a specific sound target each day.

Explanations to parents, school staff and patients

The benefit of giving detailed explanations and demonstrations to parents and carers cannot be overestimated. With a greater understanding of the aims of therapy, they are better able to carry out their part of the programme. It is recommended that the therapist observes the parent undertaking the therapy homework task to ensure correct implementation. Explanations to school staff are also important and it is essential that the therapist checks that the person supporting the child's practice understands the task and is able to recognise correct productions.

The child is also better able to participate in therapy and may be more motivated to practise if he understands the aims of therapy. Russell and Sell (1998) describe how using a cognitive approach contributed to successful therapy in older patients in the GOS-CLAPA Therapy Project. A cognitive approach means that the objectives and strategies of therapy are made explicit to the clients so that they have a full understanding of what is being done and why. For example, older children respond to detailed explanation about how consonants are produced. This includes discussion about articulatory placement and manner of articulation accompanied by diagrams and explanation.

Children can be encouraged to provide their own analogies about the aims of therapy. For younger children the concept of a 'naughty' tongue or the idea of 'training' their tongue can be useful. The language and vocabulary used should be adapted to the age of the child, but even younger clients quickly grasp the idea of teaching their tongue and lips new activities. This may be supplemented by use of the *Metaphon* concepts (Howell & Dean, 1994) and may also be aided by verbal, visual and tactile cues as described above in Chapter 5.

Audio and video feedback

Home practice can also be effectively supported with the use of audio and video tapes. As Russell and Harding (2001) comment, video tapes of modelled activities are effective in helping parents to implement a programme. They remind parents of precise modelling activities, for example, and children can reabsorb the therapist's model. Such tapes, therefore, extend the therapeutic process into the home. For older children and adult clients audio and video tapes provide feedback for their self-monitoring.

Reward systems/motivation

The general principles involved in setting up reward systems have been described above in Chapter 2, in relation to factors that influence therapy outcomes.

Young children require immediate rewards during therapy and enjoy winning stickers or items in a game; for example, monkeys to hang on the tree in the Monkey Game, or the 'swords' to push into the barrel for 'Pop-up Pirate' or similar games. As Golding-Kushner (2001) points out, the reward can be given for every response at first, but in later sessions the reward can be given after more (for example, five) correct responses. The reward should immediately follow the desired response so that the correct behaviour is reinforced. Appropriate verbal feedback is also always used with the reward system and should be given in positive terms, for example – 'Good talking', 'That's great', Good /t/ and 'Good try' with no reference being made to whether the production is right or wrong. For home practice activities, parents may use similar direct rewards.

Older children, however, may need a more sophisticated approach, perhaps working on a points or star chart system to achieve a specific goal. Regular practice can seem boring and hard work, but if they continue to have a specific goal in mind their focus is switched to achievement rather than the nature of the task. Identification of the goal needs to be given some thought. It must be realistic, achievable and, of course, motivating for the child. Russell and Sell (1998) describe how nine-year-old Nicky was prepared to work for points that would help him to achieve a specific sum of money (at a level his mother could afford). Points were awarded for daily practice, effort in therapy sessions, appropriate use of consonant targets in specific conversational situations and similar activities. This system helped Nicky to maintain his improved speech pattern. Some months after ceasing regular therapy, his mother commented that they still used the points reward system. However, each time there was a new goal, Nicky was required to put in more effort to achieve it. It therefore continued to be an effective method of supporting his speech work.

Although money worked as a goal for this particular parent and child it might be more appropriate to identify specific items, such as a comic, CD, toy or game, an outing to a particular place, or an item of clothing. A reward should not be expensive, but rather something simple that the child looks forward to and enjoys. Food items are not usually good rewards, particularly sweets, which incur displeasure from our dental colleagues! However, when this was pointed out to the mother of four-year-old Hannah, she changed the post-session reward to a piece of fruit! Fortunately Hannah liked fruit and was happy to accept this. Parents also need to understand that the promise of particular meals for being good in sessions is not likely to be effective. This is not an *immediate* reward, and the meal is usually provided anyway so it is not a true reward for effort.

Working with Teenagers and Adults

Adult clients can make changes to their speech patterns even after years of incorrect consonant production. However, as acknowledged above, they need to be highly motivated and strongly committed to put in the time and effort to achieve change. The therapist needs to investigate the reasons why an adult client has sought therapy and to understand his motivation.

Motivation and priorities

Jeremy (personal communication) reports that often the trigger for an adult client to want to work on his speech is a change in life circumstances. Here are some examples.

- A client with an unrepaired palate moved to England from Pakistan. He was assessed in an adult cleft palate clinic, had a surgical repair of the palate and was then offered therapy.
- A man, known as Jack, realised that his speech was preventing him from advancing his job prospects and getting the type of job he wanted.
- A lady with young children was concerned that they would copy her speech pattern.
- An older lady in her late sixties, and living on her own, just wanted to be understood when she gave her address. This involved production of /k/ in particular and after a few sessions she was able to 'retrieve' and use this consonant when she wanted to.

Sometimes speech is a lower priority for adult clients and is secondary to concerns about their appearance. Russell and Sell (1998) report the case of a 22-year-old student who hoped to train as a teacher and still had difficulty with /s/, which was often produced as an active nasal fricative. She was able to change her articulation and made good progress in the short term. However, the focus of her attention seemed to change from her speech to her appearance and she did not seem prepared to make the effort needed to maintain her improved speech pattern. Effectively, she lost the motivation that had moved her to seek help from a speech and language therapist.

Adult clients often face particular difficulties when they reveal to their partners, families or friends that they are seeking to make changes to their speech. These people find it difficult to understand why the client wants to change and seek to reassure him that he is fine as he is. It seems as if they do not want to offend him. This is of course in direct contrast to the response that the client may have experienced as a teenager when it seemed as if everyone was 'nagging' him about his speech!

Recognising and using improved speech

Many older children and adults find it difficult to accept that any change they achieve in their speech is an improvement and often comment that it sounds odd to them. They therefore need back up and reassurance from someone close to them that they sound better. However, they may still be reluctant to use their improved speech patterns in different situations. The client Jack, mentioned in the bullet list above, had been able to use his improved speech pattern for a long time before summoning up the courage to use it in conversation with his wife (Jeremy, personal communication). In such cases, video and audio feedback may be particularly helpful. In addition, listening to and commenting on the speech patterns of 'good' speakers and identifying what makes them sound good is also useful. For teenagers this may be someone in the public eye that they particularly admire.

The therapy programme involves the therapist and client working in partnership on agreed goals. It is a direct articulatory approach with extensive discussion regarding therapy targets and methods of consonant production, supported by audio and video feedback. EPG may be the preferred therapy method for some of these clients, particularly in cases where speech sounds distinctly 'cleft-like' because of palatalisation or lateralisation.

Checklist for therapy with teenagers and adults

1   Establish that speech work is a priority and explore motivation to change. For teenagers, a reward system may be required, as for children.
2   Discuss and agree specific aims of therapy and identify particular targets.
3   Explore how support and feedback can be provided.
4   Include an explanation of the mechanics of speech sound production in therapy.
5   Compare and contrast the speech patterns of others with the client's habitual speech production.
6   When correct articulation is achieved, maintain it in words by saying them slowly and then at speed.
7   Practise in controlled situations before attempting generalisation in other conversational contexts.

It may also help these clients if they can be introduced to others who have faced or are facing similar challenges. This can often be facilitated by the therapists working in the specialist cleft palate centres, who may arrange a group discussion session.

Appendixes

Home programme for younger children

Aims

The activities that follow aim to:

- encourage a wider range of speech-like sounds and to encourage your child to 'experiment' with his or her tongue and lip movements
- encourage copying – general and speech-like
- promote the development of listening skills
- increase mouth awareness and to encourage the use of air from the mouth for 'speech.'

The activity suggestions given are ideas which you can select from and incorporate into your child's daily routine. They all connect to each other and can, therefore, be mixed. Use opportunities that present naturally to carry out some of the activities. Involve brothers and/or sisters and others. Please remember that all the activities should be presented as a game, not as a task. They should be relaxed, fun and not cause stress for your child apart from learning to listen and respond appropriately. Have fun!

Babble sessions

Participative babble sessions

Start by practising with your child those strings of sounds that he or she can achieve easily, for example _____ (to be filled in by speech and language therapist). Then move on to other easier ones, for example _____

Vary the vowel sounds you use (ay, ee, eye, oh, etc). Also vary your volume, making some sounds quietly and others louder. Make the tone of your voice go up and down. During these sessions, let your child feel your face and lips and also his or her own. Perhaps babble against different parts of the body. Some people find that there are particularly good times of day when their children seem especially communicative (for example, bathtime or changing time) and these are the best times for babble sessions.

This page may be photocopied for instructional use only. *Practical Intervention for Cleft Palate Speech* © Jane Russell & Liz Albery 2005

Routledge Taylor & Francis Group

Practical Intervention for Cleft Palate Speech © Jane Russell & Liz Albery 2005

Routledge
Taylor & Francis Group

Using games to show different tones of voice

When swinging your child or bouncing him or her up and down on your lap, make your voice go up and down as you say 'up' and 'down'. When your child imitates the rising and falling pattern of your voice in his or her vocalising, keep repeating the activity to encourage him or her to continue. Use the pitch of your voice and your inflection to communicate emotions such as joy, anger or surprise. You will perhaps need to over-emphasise these to start with.

Singing songs and nursery rhymes

Sing simple songs and rhymes to your child and encourage him or her to join in with the melody and the words. Such rhymes include those accompanied by hand actions, for example, 'Round and round the garden' and 'This little piggy'.

Everyday sounds and noises

Look for opportunities during play and daily activities to associate particular sounds with objects and actions. For example, 't, t, t' with a dripping tap and a prolonged 'sh' associated with washing the car, or a fireman using a hose. Remember to make sure that the sounds you use are speech-like sounds and in particular *do not* use or repeat 'growls' made at the back of the throat. Respond to such vocalisations from your child by using a different and more speech-like sound.

Copying

Whole-body movements

Some of these activities can be carried out in front of a mirror. Use a full length mirror for the whole-body movements. Encourage your child to copy whole-body movements, such as clapping, dancing, jumping and waving the arms up and down. Make the game slightly harder as the child achieves success and add copying of mimed activities such as brushing your teeth or washing your face. During this, you should comment using the right words so that your child also learns new words and language. Older children will enjoy a 'Simon says' game. This is also a good game for other children and adults to join in.

Face, tongue and lip movements

Move on to copying face movements, such as smiling, frowning, yawning and blinking. Make faces at each other in the mirror and use 'oo' and 'ah' sounds with different facial expressions. From this you can move on to copying tongue and lip movements. This copying activity links with the babbling practice described above. Encourage your child to copy different lip shapes, associating the shapes with specific objects or actions, for example, 'o' with a fish. For tongue movements, show your child how you put your tongue out and then pull it back into your mouth and close your lips. Repeat this action several times. Then you can teach him or her how to move the tongue from side to side and up and down outside the mouth.

Listening

Identifying different sound makers

Use different sound makers, such as a whistle, bell or rattle. Use some of your child's toys and some other items (such as a spoon in a cup). Show your child which object makes which sound. Ask him or her to find the one that he or she hears when you have hidden it behind a cover or box, for example.

Listening for the hidden object

Hide a toy that makes a noise when it is wound up, or a ticking clock, and see if your child can find it. You can also associate the noise with a speech sound like 't' or 'k', as in the babbling practice.

Following whispered instructions

Play games in which your child has to follow whispered instructions to do something or find a picture or toy. Encourage your child and others playing the game to take their turn at being the one to tell the others what to do. Use audiotapes of familiar songs and rhymes. Turn the volume very low and see if your child can guess which song it is.

Mouth awareness and mouth airstream

Encourage the lip smacking and 'blowing raspberries' sounds that babies make naturally and also the sounds that occur when a finger is stroked against the lips while vocalising. Let your child feel how air from your mouth feels against his or her hand

Practical Intervention for Cleft Palate Speech © Jane Russell & Liz Albery 2005

Routledge
Taylor & Francis Group

when you blow very gently. Gently blow to cool hot food in real or pretend situations. Holding your child's nose gently while he or she attempts to blow might help the child to experience the right sensation. These actions *must* be relaxed and gentle. Stop if you think that your child is trying too hard.

When your child has some success with gentle blowing, start to associate this with speech-like sounds; for example, adding the lip and teeth position for 'f' or making a bubble on a wand 'wobble' when you say 'p, p, p'.

Remember: this is all a game. Have fun playing with your child!

Routledge
Taylor & Francis Group

Home Diary

2

Name

Date

Today we have worked on the sound/s:

Please could you practise these with

A short session everyday is helpful, even if it's only for 10 minutes. Please note down any problems with the practice sounds so that we can discuss them at the next session which is on

at   . Thank you!

Routledge
Taylor & Francis Group

3 Advice for teachers

Cleft lip and/or palate affects about one in 700 of the population. Children who have a cleft lip only usually have no problem with speech, but a cleft palate can affect speech. There are different combinations of cleft lip and palate, as shown below.

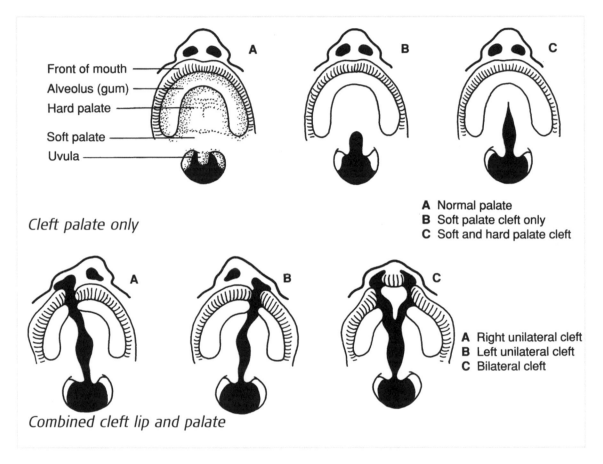

Front of mouth
Alveolus (gum)
Hard palate
Soft palate
Uvula

Cleft palate only

A Normal palate
B Soft palate cleft only
C Soft and hard palate cleft

A Right unilateral cleft
B Left unilateral cleft
C Bilateral cleft

Combined cleft lip and palate

The surgery for repair of cleft lip and palate usually takes place in a hospital specialising in this surgery, during the first year of a child's life. More operations may be necessary as the child grows, including further surgery to help speech. Around 50 per cent of children with cleft palate need speech therapy.

Speech & Language Therapy

If a child has a cleft palate, his or her speech should be assessed regularly by the specialist speech and language therapist who works as part of the cleft palate team in the hospital where the child's surgery has taken place. Any therapy needed is often the responsibility of the child's local speech and language therapist, who will see the child in school or at the local health centre. Each child should have an individual therapy programme and it is helpful if the therapist can liaise with you so that you know, for example, what sound/s the child is working on. It is very helpful to the child's progress if you can reinforce (time permitting!) the work that the speech and language therapist is doing, in class activities. For example, you might give one-to-one reading practice and provide gentle reminders of a correct sound when the child is talking directly to you. Obviously, correcting a child in front of the class is not helpful and may be demotivating.

Hearing

Most children with a cleft palate have a fluctuating hearing loss and are more prone to ear infections than children without a cleft. In some cases, small tubes (grommets) may need to be inserted in the ear by an ear, nose and throat surgeon, or the child may need to wear hearing aids. Teachers need to be aware of the possibility of hearing loss in a child with a cleft palate and check that any hearing difficulty is being followed up in a clinic. If there is evidence of hearing loss it is helpful, if possible, to position a child close to the teacher in the classroom and to face the child and speak clearly when talking one-to-one.

Hospitalisation

The number of operations needed for a child with a cleft lip and palate varies but it is quite likely that some schooling will be missed during periods of time in hospital, or for outpatient appointments. If there is any concern about a child falling behind at school, many hospitals have teachers available who are pleased to supervise any work sent with a child coming into hospital. Some children positively enjoy the experience of going into hospital, while for others it is a major trauma. It is best if children are told of hospital admission, and what to expect, in a simple and truthful way.

Behaviour of peers

It is quite common for children with cleft lip and palate to be teased at school by their peers. Typically this behaviour starts at around seven or eight years of age and can continue until a child leaves school. It is often very distressing for the child and his or her parents, and it is not always possible to eradicate it completely. The teacher has a role here in being sensitive to the possibility of teasing and, if it occurs, in helping to deal with it. This may involve talking to the 'victim' and the perpetrators and all the parents concerned or bringing into play the school's protocol for bullying. One mother of a child who had been teased went into school to give a talk on cleft lip and palate, which proved successful. However, different situations, cultures and personalities demand different solutions. A particular problem can be referred to the cleft palate team, who should have the services of a clinical psychologist to advise the child and parents on ways in which to deal with teasing.

4 Resources

1 Therapy Materials

Big Mouth Sound Pack
STASS Publications
44 North Road
Ponteland
Northumberland
NE20 9UR
UK
Tel. 01661 822316
www.stasspublications.co.uk

Black Sheep Consonant Worksheets
Black Sheep Press
67 Middleton
Cowling
Keighley
West Yorks
BD22 0DQ
UK
Tel. 01535 631346
www.blacksheep-epress.com

Clapa Thameside Games
Speech and Language Therapy Department
St Andrew's Centre for Plastic Surgery
Broomfield Hospital
Court Road
Broomfield
Chelmsford
CM1 7ET
UK
Tel. 01245 516020

GOS-CLAPA
GOS-CLAPA Video – Speech Assessment
(GOS.SP.ASS '94 &'98) – A Training Video of
Speech Characteristics

The GOS-CLAPA Therapy Project Video –
Principles and Techniques of Speech Therapy
Treatment

Both available from:
Department of Medical Illustration
Great Ormond Street Hospital
Great Ormond Street
London
WC1N 3JH
UK
Tel: 020 7829 7895

Jolly Learning Ltd
Tailours House
High Road
Chigwell
Essex
IG7 6DL
UK
www.jollylearning.co.uk

The Mighty Mouth Board Game
Super Duper Publications
POBox 24997
Greenville SC 29616
USA
www.superduperinc.com
or
Winslow
Goytside Road
Chesterfield
Derbyshire
S40 2PH
UK
www.winslow-cat.com

MSIM
The Use of Multi-Sensory Input Modelling to Stimulate Speech Output Processing –
A Demonstration Video (Harding-Bell & Bryan, 2003).

Available from:
Anne Harding-Bell
Lead Specialist Speech & Language Therapist
Dept of Plastic & Reconstructive Surgery
Box 46
Addenbrookes Hospital,
Hills Road
Cambridge
CB2 2QQ
UK

Mr Tongue
SLT Department
Dudley South PCT
The Speech Centre
Central Clinic
Hall Street
Dudley
DY2 7BX
UK

Nuffield Centre Dyspraxia Programme
The Principal Speech and Language Therapist
Nuffield Hearing and Speech Centre
Royal National Throat, Nose and Ear Hospital
330 Gray's Inn Road
London
WC1X 8DA
UK

2 Computer-assisted Therapy

For reviews of suitable software applications please visit **www.speech-therapy.org**

Articulation 1,11 &111
Locotour Multimedia
(Learning Fundamentals)
1130 Grove Street
Suite 300
San Luis Obispo
CA 93401, USA
www.locutour.com

Electropalatography (EPG)
Articulate Instruments
Queen Margaret Campus
36 Clerwood Terrace
Edinburgh EH128TS
Scotland

Speech Sounds on Cue
Propeller Multimedia Limited
PO Box 27028
Edinburgh EH10 6WD
Scotland
Tel 0131 446 0820
www.propeller.net

Speech Viewer III
IBM UK Ltd
PO Box 41
North Harbour
Portsmouth
Hampshire PO6 3AU
UK
Tel 01475 892000
www.ibm.com/ibm/uk

3 Useful Websites

www.clapa.com (Cleft Lip and Palate Association)
A number of useful publications for parents and professionals are available from this site.

www.vcfsef.org (VCFS Educational Foundation)

www.maxappeal.org.uk
Provides family support for 22q11 deletion.

www.cleftSLTSIG.org
Website for speech and language therapists with a special interest in cleft lip and palate/craniofacial disorders and velopharyngeal dysfunction.

Bibliography

Albery EH & Enderby P, 1984, 'Intensive Therapy for Cleft Palate Children', *British Journal of Disorders of Communication* 19, pp115–24.

Albery EH, Hathorn IS & Pigott RW, 1986, *Cleft Lip and Palate: A Team Approach*, Churchill Livingstone, London.

Albery EH & Russell J, 1990, 'Cleft Palate and Orofacial Abnormalities', Grunwell P (ed), *Developmental Speech Disorders*, Churchill Livingstone, London.

Bamford J & Saunders E, 1990, *Hearing Impairment, Auditory Perception and Language Disability*, 2nd edn, Whurr, London.

Clinical Standards Advisory Group, 1998, *Cleft Lip and/or Palate*, The Stationery Office, London.

Dodd B, 1995, 'A Problem Solving Approach to Clinical Management', Dodd B (ed), *Differential Diagnosis and Treatment of Children with Speech Disorders*, Whurr, London.

Golding-Kushner KJ, 1995, 'Treatment of Articulation and Resonance Disorders Associated with Cleft Palate and VPI', Shprintzen RJ, Bardach J (eds), *Cleft Palate Speech Management: A Multidisciplinary Approach to the Management of Cleft Palate*, CV Mosby, St Louis.

Golding-Kushner KJ, 2001, *Therapy Techniques for Cleft Palate Speech & Related Disorders*, Singular, San Diego.

Grundy K & Harding A, 1995, 'Disorders of Speech Production', Grundy K (ed), *Linguistics in Clinical Practice*, 2nd edn, Taylor & Francis, London.

Grunwell P, 1985, *Phonological Assessment of Child Speech (PACS)*, NFER-Nelson, Windsor.

Grunwell P, 1993, *Analysing Cleft Palate Speech*, Whurr, London.

Grunwell P & Dive D, 1988, 'Treating Cleft Palate Speech', *Child Language Teaching and Therapy* 4, pp193–210.

Harding A & Grunwell P, 1998, 'Active versus Passive Cleft-type Speech Characteristics', *International Journal of Disorders of Communication and Language*, 33, pp329–52.

Harding-Bell A & Bryan, 2003, *The Use of Multi-Sensory Input Modelling to Stimulate Speech Output Processing – a Demonstration Video*.

Hoch L, Golding-Kushner KJ, Siegel-Sadewitz VL & Shprintzen RJ, 1986, Speech Therapy, *Seminars in Speech and Language* 7, pp311–23.

Howell J & Dean E, 1994, *Treating Phonological Disorders in Children, Metaphon – Theory to Practice*, 2nd edn, Whurr, London.

Jeremy A, 2000, Personal communication.

John A, Sell D, Harding-Bell A, Sweeney T & Williams A, in press, 'CAPS-A: A Validated and Reliable Measure for Auditing Cleft Palate Speech', *Cleft Palate – Craniofacial Journal.*

Le Blanc EM, 1996, 'Fundamental Principles in the Speech Management of Cleft Lip and Palate', Berkowitz S (ed), *Cleft Lip and Palate: Perspectives in Management. Vol 2 An Introduction to Craniofacial Anomalies*, Singular Publishing, San Diego.

Lennox P, 2001, 'Hearing and ENT Management', Watson A, Sell D & Grunwell P (eds), *Management of Cleft Lip and Palate,* Whurr, London.

McWilliams BJ, Morris HL & Shelton RL, 1990, *Cleft Palate Speech*, 2nd edn, B C Decker, Philadelphia.

Morley ME, 1970, *Cleft Palate and Speech*, 7th edn. Williams & Wilkins, Baltimore.

Nuffield Speech & Hearing Centre, 1985, 1992, *Nuffield Centre Dyspraxia Programme.*

Passy J, 1990, *Cued Articulation*, STASS Publications, Ponteland.

Russell VJ, 1989, 'Early Intervention', Stengelhofen J (ed), *Cleft Palate: The Nature and Remediation of Communication Problems*, Churchill Livingstone, London.

Russell J, 1997, 'The Timing of Consonant Articulation Therapy in Relation to Velopharyngeal Surgery', Paper presented at Craniofacial Society of Great Britain Annual Scientific Conference, Writtle, Essex.

Russell J & Grunwell P, 1993, 'Speech Development in Children with Cleft Lip and Palate', Grunwell P (ed), *Analysing Cleft Palate Speech*, Whurr, London.

Russell VJ & Harding A, 2001, 'Speech Development and Early Intervention', Watson A, Sell D & Grunwell P (eds), *Cleft Palate Management*, Whurr, London.

Russell J & Sell D, 1998, *The GOS-CLAPA Therapy Project – Principles and Techniques of Speech Therapy Treatment*, Department of Medical Illustration, Great Ormond Street Hospital, Great Ormond Street, London WC1N 3JH.

Sell D & Grunwell P, 1993, 'Speech in Subjects with Late Operated Cleft Palate', Grunwell P (ed), *Analysing Cleft Palate Speech*, Whurr, London.

Sell D & Grunwell P, 2001, 'Speech Assessment and Therapy', Watson A, Sell D & Grunwell P (eds), *Cleft Palate Management*, Whurr, London.

Sell D, Harding A & Grunwell P, 1994, 'A Screening Assessment of Cleft Palate Speech: GOS.SP.ASS (Great Ormond Street Speech Assessment)', *European Journal of Disorders of Communication* 28, pp1–15.

Sell D, Harding A & Grunwell P, 1999, Revised GOS.SP.ASS (98): Speech Assessment For Children With Cleft Palate And/Or Velopharyngeal Dysfunction (Revised)', *International Journal of Disorders of Communication* 34, pp17–33.

Stark RE, 1986, 'Prespeech Segmental Feature Development', Fletcher P & Garman M (eds), *Language Acquisition,* 2nd edn, University Press, Cambridge.

Stengelhofen J, 1990, *Working with Cleft Palate,* Winslow Press, Bicester.

Stoel-Gammon C, 1992, 'Prelinguistic Vocal Development', Ferguson C, Menn L & Stoel-Gammon (eds), *Phonological Development, Models, Research, Implications,* York Press, Maryland.

Van Demark DR & Hardin MA, 1990, 'Speech Therapy for the Child with Cleft Lip and Palate', Bardach J & Morris HL (eds), *Multidisciplinary Management of Cleft Lip and Palate,* Saunders, Philadelphia.

Watson A, Sell D & Grunwell P, 2001, *Cleft Palate Management,* Whurr, London.

9 780863 885136

9780863885136

T - #0004 - 290721 - C0 - 297/210/7 - SB - 9780863885136 - Gloss Lamination